COMPUTERIZING
A CLINICAL LABORATORY

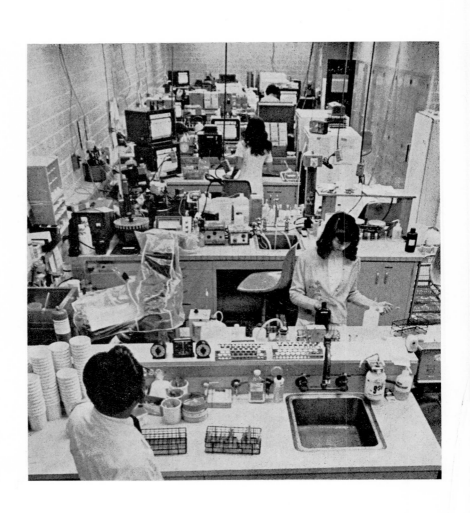

Computerizing

A Clinical

Laboratory

By

JERRY K. AIKAWA, M.D.

Professor of Medicine
Director, Laboratory Services
Director, Allied Health Programs
University of Colorado Medical Center
Denver, Colorado

and

EDWARD R. PINFIELD

Instructor of Medicine
Laboratory Computer Systems Designer
University of Colorado Medical Center
Denver, Colorado

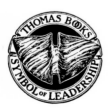

CHARLES C THOMAS · PUBLISHER
Springfield · Illinois · U.S.A.

Published and Distributed Throughout the World by
CHARLES C THOMAS • PUBLISHER
BANNERSTONE HOUSE
301-327 East Lawrence Avenue, Springfield, Illinois, U.S.A.

© *1973, by* CHARLES C THOMAS • PUBLISHER
ISBN 0-398-02847-8
Library of Congress Catalog Card Number: 73-5661

With THOMAS BOOKS *careful attention is given to all details of manufacturing and design. It is the Publisher's desire to present books that are satisfactory as to their physical qualities and artistic possibilities and appropriate for their particular use.* THOMAS BOOKS *will be true to those laws of quality that assure a good name and good will.*

Library of Congress Cataloging in Publication Data

Aikawa, Jerry Kazuo, 1921-
    Computerizing a clinical laboratory.

    1. Electronic data processing—Clinical medicine. I. Pinfield, Edward R., joint author. II. Title. [DNLM: 1. Computers. 2. Diagnosis, Laboratory. QY 26.5 A291c 1973]
RB38.A34   616'.0028'54   73-5661
ISBN 0-398-02847-8

Printed in the United States of America
N-1

Dedicated
to
The Central Laboratory Staff

Debit	*Credit*
Sometimes chauvinistic	Usually accurate
disgruntled	courteous
emotional	efficient
obstinate	friendly
temperamental	neat
	punctual
	In the balance,

A GEM

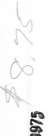

PREFACE

W HEN FIRST I ANNOUNCED to the staff that *we* were going to write a book about the computerization of our laboratory, one member exclaimed, "Who on earth would bother to buy, much less to read, such a book!" The reaction might have been anticipated—to them the computer is a way of life. Besides, it is not respectable in our medical center setting to be so concerned about improvement in the delivery of health care.

At a time when basic scientists are retreating further behind membranes and the public is clamoring for expanded health care as a God-given right, the health care system (if indeed it is a system) is becoming increasingly clogged with information which it cannot digest, store, or transfer. More than twenty-five percent of the hospital budget may be spent for information processing;[1] yet the information glut continues.

There is a logical solution to the dilemma: it is to computerize, to merge the management information system with an embryonic data processing system, such as that in the clinical laboratory, as the nucleus for a single clinical data processing system. Several years ago the giant of the industry attempted to swallow a total hospital information system, required gavage, and in the process created countless skeptics. Who then will supply the enthusiasm, the will, and the manpower to design and implement such a system? Certainly in our setting the laboratory will be a major contributor.

This book is intended for every laboratory director who has thought seriously about using the computer to improve the quality of health care and delivery. It is intended also for clinicians who are interested in the same subject, because the clinical data processing system will not evolve unless they become involved in this mammoth project.

[1]R.A. Jydstrum, and Gross, M.J.: Cost of information handling in hospitals. *Health Serv Res, 1*:235-271, 1966.

We have all been led to believe that the development of a data processing system is something mysterious, restricted to computer experts. One of the purposes of writing this book is to prove that this is not the case. We do not claim to be experts. We merely wish to testify that amateurs can build computer systems which work. As a matter of fact, computer experts oftentimes get in the way.

Our highly automated and computerized clinical laboratory system has expanded since the initial segment went *on-line* in October, 1968, and continues to grow. In the process of developing this system, we have committed many errors out of sheer abysmal ignorance. We hope that the reader will profit from them as much as from our successes.

This is the story of how the University of Colorado clinical laboratory computer system came to be.

ACKNOWLEDGMENTS

A LABORATORY COMPUTER SYSTEM cannot be developed without the enthusiastic support and plain hard work of a devoted team of workers. We wish to express our appreciation and gratitude to the following individuals:

From IBM:
 Eldon C. Johnsen
 Don Johnson
 Ruth Mossman
 Mary Jane Stevens
 Warren T. Stuart

From the Medical Center Administration:
 Don L. Arnwine
 Charles J. Austin
 George S. Tyner, M.D.

From the Central Laboratory Staff:
 Carl R. Ashwood
 Carol Augspurger
 Richard N. Camfield
 Daniel Cooper
 Alberta P. David
 K. Patricia DeChaney
 Dale R. Harms
 Arlin E. James
 Edna E. Mains
 Roy H. Ott, M.D.
 J. Richard Pearson, Ph.D.
 Arnold Takemoto

Our thanks go to Mrs. Junioretta Zimmerman for her excellent secretarial help and to Mrs. Alberta David for her editorial assistance.

CONTENTS

COMPUTERIZING
A CLINICAL LABORATORY

● ●

CHAPTER 1

INTRODUCTION

A LEGACY

"**A** KITCHEN TABLE, with a few shelves for bottles, screened off in a corner of the office, will suffice for a laboratory."[2] So wrote in 1908 Dr. James Campbell Todd, Associate Professor of Pathology at the University of Colorado School of Medicine and author of the oldest, continuously published American textbook of clinical pathology.[3] If Dr. Todd were here today, he would probably admonish us for our extravagances. Dr. Robert C. Lewis, Professor of Biochemistry and former Dean of the University of Colorado School of Medicine, was senior author with Dr. Stanley R. Benedict of the report describing the first practical analytic method for blood glucose.[4] Dr. Lewis could scarcely have predicted that automated equipment would be performing scores of chemical analyses hourly with minimal human intervention. It must be apparent to the reader that since its founding this University has contributed much to a proud tradition in Laboratory Medicine. And history has given us an opportunity to continue in the footsteps of these pioneers.

EARLY HISTORY

The University of Colorado Medical Center at 4200 East Ninth Avenue, Denver, Colorado, was a product of the reform in medical education which reverberated across the continent fol-

---

[2]James C. Todd: *A Syllabus of Lectures Upon Clinical Diagnosis.* 1906-1907. Reprinted from Denver Medical Times and Utah Medical Journal.

[3]James C. Todd: *A Manual of Clinical Diagnosis.* Philadelphia, Saunders, 1908.

[4]R.C. Lewis, and Benedict, S.R.: A method for the estimation of sugar in small quantities of blood. *Proc Soc Exper Biol Med, 11:*57-58, 1913.

3

lowing the Flexner report.[5] The new Colorado General Hospital opened in September, 1924, and the University of Colorado School of Medicine adopted a four year curriculum with a prerequisite of at least three years of college preparatory work.

Dr. Todd has been credited with being the first medical educator to advocate a chair for Clinical Pathology in medical schools. At his request, a separate Department of Clinical Pathology was created in 1916 at the University of Colorado School of Medicine. Dr. Edward R. Mugrage, a protégé of Dr. Todd, was professor and head of this department from 1916 until his retirement in 1953. This department was responsible primarily for routine hematologic analyses, urinalyses, and simple serologic assays. Biochemical and microbiologic assays which were required for patient care were performed reluctantly by the basic science departments of Biochemistry and Microbiology. It was essentially a Monday through Friday, 8 a.m. to 5 p.m. service, with emergency calls taken by eager but sometimes poorly qualified graduate students.

REORGANIZATION

Upon Dr. Mugrage's retirement in 1953, the Department of Clinical Pathology became a Division within the Department of Medicine and a consolidated authority was established for a centralized laboratory facility at the Medical Center. Hematology, Microbiology, and Clinical Chemistry thus became sections of the Central Laboratory. Dr. Joseph H. Holmes, Professor of Medicine, was appointed Director of the Central Laboratory and held this position from 1953 until 1958.

PERIOD OF STATUS QUO

Although some would take issue with this generalization, from the 1920's through the early 1940's nothing much new developed in clinical laboratories. Most laboratories were makeshift affairs, likely as not located in a closet or in the basement of the hospital.

[5]Abraham Flexner: *Medical Education in the United States and Canada. A Report to the Carnegie Foundation for the Advancement of Teaching.* Boston, Merrymont Press, 1910.

Hematology was performed in the traditional manner. The repertoire in clinical chemistry remained limited and essentially stable, and microbiology was an art of limited clinical applicability. Laboratory information was considered *ancillary* to the clinical history and the physical examination. That is to say, the clinician was happy when the laboratory data confirmed his clinical impression but disregarded the information when it did not. After all, the laboratory was not that reliable! These were the years when the clinical laboratory was a stepchild of anatomic pathology.

From the mid-1940's onward, a refreshing breeze replaced the stagnation in the hospital laboratory. Photoelectric spectrophotometers replaced visual colorimeters. Controlled temperature heating baths replaced coffee cans. Flame photometers reached the hospital laboratory. The availability of antibiotics transformed bacteriology into an applied science. Radioisotopes became available in quantity and at a reasonable cost. The Federal Government began investing heavily in medical research.

During this period the laboratory began to be faced with serious problems of the increasing cost of supplies and specialized equipment, the shortage of trained personnel, inadequate space, and the increasing demand for services. The solution, however, was not in sight as long as the analyses were performed manually by the classic methods.

INTRODUCTION OF AUTOMATION

Changes in methods were necessary for the survival of the laboratory. At first, attempts were made to modify classic glassware, such as burets and pipets.[6] Some of these were semiautomated so that, by flipping a lever, a motor driven buret or pipet would deliver repetitively the same volume of fluid from a single container. A different concept involving more complete automation was introduced during the same period in the early 1950's. Dr. Leonard T. Skeggs devised an instrument which sequentially and automatically analyzed chemical components of blood in a

---

[6]J.K. Aikawa, Reardon, J.Z., and Plym, A.: An automated diluting buret. *Am J Clin Path,* 39:326-327, 1963.

closed system using air bubbles to separate discrete samples.[7] This continuous flow system was marketed under the trade name Auto-Analyzer by the Technicon Corporation. Whereas in the past a medical technologist was able to perform manually only forty to sixty determinations per day, the AutoAnalyzer analyzed at the rate of forty to sixty per hour. If the sample stream were divided into two, four, or greater numbers of separate parallel channels, simultaneous analyses could be performed for any number of chemical constituents.

The Central Laboratory acquired its first AutoAnalyzer in 1957 at a cost of $3,000. A resident in Clinical Pathology was assigned the responsibility of setting up an automated method for glucose. In retrospect there was inadequate instruction of the technical staff in the theory, the operation, and the maintenance of the equipment; this failure in management resulted in skepticism, resentment, and resistance to change. (It is of historic interest that in the same year the laboratory spent $335 for a Mc-Kesson BMR machine as a replacement for another unit which was sixteen years old.)

On March 17, 1958, automated analyses of glucose and blood urea nitrogen (BUN) were offered daily for the first time. These analyses were *batch-processed,* the manifold being changed to run one or the other test. The Central Laboratory acquired its second AutoAnalyzer in 1960. With only two units available, the extent of the automation amounted to a simultaneous determination of blood glucose and BUN or of alkaline phosphatase and its blank. All other analyses were performed manually.

By 1958 the Central Laboratory was experiencing a progressive annual increment of 15-20 percent in work load. Further automation was necessary for survival. The Annual Report of the Central Laboratory for fiscal year 1958-1959 recognized this problem:

> "Our objective continues to be to provide the most efficient, comprehensive, and reliable laboratory service at the lowest possible cost. The largest single item in the budget is the salary of medical technologists. Any method for reducing technical time will reduce cost appreciably. It is for this reason that we are extremely interested in

---

[7]L.T. Skeggs, Jr.: An automatic method for colorimetric analysis. *Am J Clin Path,* *28:*311-322, 1957.

testing and adopting, when reliable, any and all automatic devices. Although the initial cost of some of this equipment is high, it should, in the long run, result in economy and greater reliability of results."

The rate of change in the introduction of automated methods increased in Clinical Chemistry between 1959 and 1964. During the fiscal year 1963-1964, the total number of tests performed was 92,025, an increase of 17.5 percent from the previous year, but the cost per test had decreased from $0.92 to $0.80. This reduction was undoubtedly a reflection of an increased efficiency of operation due to greater automation.

FURTHER AUTOMATION

Planning began in earnest in 1960 for a new Colorado General Hospital. An interested and concerned *ad hoc* committee appointed by the dean allocated 12,000 sq. ft. of floor space for a new central laboratory facility. Development of the detailed floor plans for each of the major functional areas was assigned to the supervisors of each area. The equipment budget for the new hospital provided generously for additional automated instruments. The actual move to the new facility took place smoothly over a period of twelve hours on February 19, 1965. Immediately afterwards, the Central Laboratory was performing automated determinations of BUN and creatinine, blood glucose, alkaline phosphatase, and phosphate. A few months later, with the acquisition of additional instruments, automated determinations were offered for uric acid, simultaneous sodium, potassium, chloride and carbon dioxide, and cholesterol. Thus, over 85 percent of the work in Clinical Chemistry was fully automated by June 30, 1965.

The problem of the actual performance of the chemical analytic process itself had been solved, at least in theory, by automation.

QUALITY CONTROL

At about the time that the first AutoAnalyzers were being marketed, some laboratories began to give serious thought to the problem of reproducibility and accuracy of laboratory data,[8] that is, to the subject of quality control. In a nutshell, what happened

---

[8]A. Plym, and Aikawa, J.K.: The evaluation of laboratory data by means of quality control. A programmed instruction manual. *Am J Med Tech, 32*:219-230, 1966.

was that the statistical methods and the experimental designs that were employed for years in the research laboratory finally reached the clinical laboratory. The previously prevalent attitude that certain laboratory results were *good enough* for clinical purposes was replaced by a new one which dictated that only the best, the most specific, and the most precise methods should be used in the care of patients.

On January 25, 1962, the Central Laboratory was able to report to the Dean that:

> "Statistical analysis of data has been practiced in the research laboratory for many years. Wherever applicable the methods of research are now being applied to control of the quality of results in the Central Laboratory. For the past year we have been routinely including quality control measurements in our daily runs. By analysis of the consistency of the results of control specimens, it is possible to set confidence limits for each determination. Analyses of these data suggest that automated devices give consistently more reproducible results than manual methods."

An extensive system of quality control has been in continuous operation in the Clinical Chemistry section of the Central Laboratory since 1961 (Fig. 1). Pooled bovine serum is purchased from a veterinary firm, its components adjusted, and aliquots lyophilized or frozen. Three control specimens, one each in the low, medium, and high ranges, are analyzed with each run.

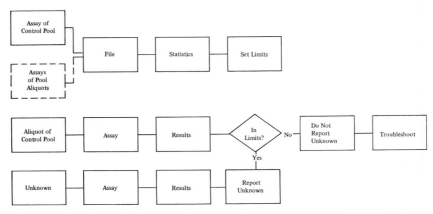

Figure 1. A schematic diagram of the quality control system which has been in use in the Central Laboratory since 1961.

●●●●●●●●●●●●●●●●●●●●●●●●●●●●

CHAPTER II

THE BEGINNING OF DATA PROCESSING

INITIAL PLANS

W E DO NOT RECALL the exact moment when we realized that automation was changing traditional concepts of the responsibilities of a clinical laboratory. The laboratory had been so busy performing the actual analyses that it had very little time to consider other matters. Only after automation had eliminated some of the manual procedures in chemistry did the staff have time to analyze the tasks which kept it so busy. It then was obvious that the clerical aspects of sample identification, calculation, interpolation, and reporting of results required up to twice as much of the technologists' time as that required by the analytic process. As analog signals poured out of AutoAnalyzers, we could no longer ignore this inappropriate expenditure of time and effort by a highly trained technical staff for clerical functions.

So it was that by the end of 1963 the laboratory staff began exploring the use of an International Business Machines Corporation (IBM) 402 unit record accounting machine. The objectives of the 402 system were (1) to assist in assembling laboratory reports and to print them in a legible form and (2) to carry on some of the business functions of the laboratory, such as the generation of charges and the accumulation of statistics. This was the mechanization of information transfer in its most elementary form, not much advanced over the system used by Dr. Herman Hollerith to process data for the 1890 Census.

By July, 1964, plans had progressed sufficiently that a purchase order was submitted to IBM for the 402 unit record system which was delivered in October. Two members of the office staff attended IBM's Customer Training sessions to learn to keypunch.

UNIT RECORD SYSTEM

Data cards measuring $3\frac{1}{4}$" x $7\frac{3}{8}$" and with provision for eighty columns of Hollerith-coded information were used to identify the tests performed and the patients on whom such tests were requested. The patient-identifying information was keypunched into one card and was merged by machine with the test information that had been prepunched in other cards. A set of such cards now contained essential information concerning the patient and the test. The laboratory used a mechanical sorting machine to reshuffle the cards according to patients or types of tests so that a *pick-up list* or a laboratory *worksheet* could be printed with the accounting machine.

After the analog signals from the AutoAnalyzers had been identified and the necessary interpolations and calculations made, the technologists wrote test results for each sample on the worksheets; each test result was keypunched into the appropriate test card. The cards, resorted according to patient, were fed into the accounting machine which printed legible laboratory reports that became the final documents for the patient's chart. In a similar fashion, all laboratory financial transactions concerning charges and credits were summarized once daily for submission to the hospital finance office. This system, flow-charted in Figure 2, became operational on April 1, 1965, and functioned very effectively. The cost to the laboratory was $384.80 per month for lease of the equipment.

This elementary system introduced our laboratory staff to the implements and language of mechanized data processing and to a more standardized and rigorous operating procedure than that to which it had been accustomed. Exposure of the staff to these elements paved the way to enlightened participation in computerization.

Any reader who is not familiar with the jargon of the computer field should refer to Appendix I.

1. Request forms received.

2. Keypunch one patient master card for each sample.

3. Pull a prepunched test card, one for each test requested. Place behind the patient master card punched at step #2.

4. Gangpunch data from patient master card into each test card.

5. Separate the patient master cards from the test cards on the sorter.

6. Sort test cards by sample No.

7. Print log sheet.

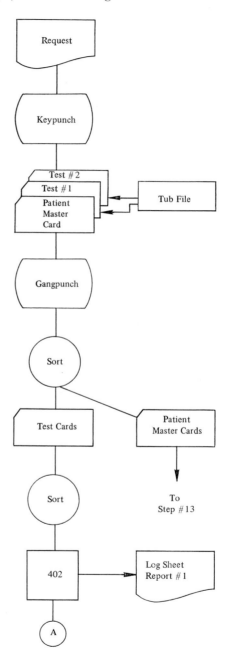

8. Sort into test number sequence.

9. Merge worksheet header cards
   in front of test cards.

10. Print worksheets. Return
    header cards to their file.
    Test cards go to step #11.

11. Punch results into test cards.

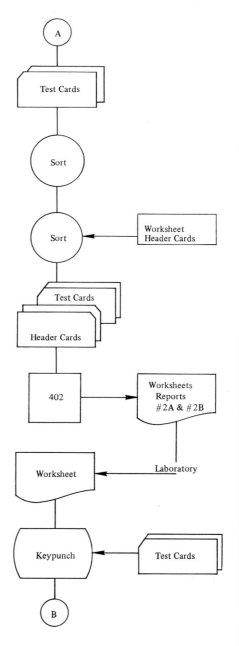

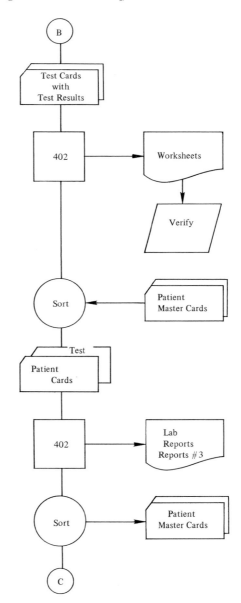

12. List punched test cards on worksheets and verify printed results against handwritten results. Correct any errors in cards.

13. Merge patient master cards from step #5.

14. Print Lab reports for patients' charts.

15. Sort to separate. File master cards. Sort test cards alphabetically by patient name.

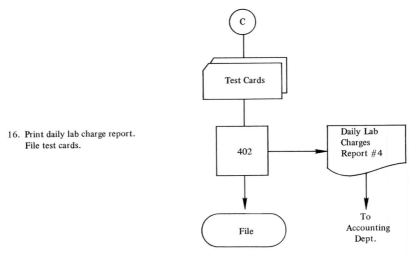

16. Print daily lab charge report.
    File test cards.

Figure 2. A flowchart of the unit record system.

CHAPTER III

PLANNING FOR A COMPUTERIZED SYSTEM

INITIAL STEPS

THE 402 SYSTEM had been operational for only a few months before a more ambitious plan was being explored. The International Business Machines Corporation (IBM) had just introduced the 1800 computer. This computer system, described as a process control monitor, is designed to record continuously analog or digital signals, to perform calibration and quality control functions, and to automatically store, retrieve, and print data. With it, we could automatically couple each line of AutoAnalyzer to the 1800 and eliminate the necessity of human intervention in many time-consuming and error-prone tasks.

In July, 1965, several major administrative decisions were made: to order the 1800 system, to subsidize all developmental costs from the operating budget of the Central Laboratory rather than through research grants, and to encourage total involvement of the laboratory staff in this endeavor. We were committed, thereby, to the development of a unique laboratory system based on faith that the eventual financial benefits and the improvements in efficiency, accuracy, and speed would justify the tremendous financial outlay. The 1800 was scheduled for delivery in September, 1966.

OBJECTIVES OF THE LABORATORY SYSTEM

The *objectives of the laboratory system* as originally planned were:

(1) to reduce the amount of clerical work performed by the medical technologist,

(2) to minimize transcription errors,

(3) to utilize the potential of a process control monitor in linking mechanization to computerization,

(4) to incorporate a quality control mechanism in the system,

(5) to return a written report to the physician as soon as possible after the analytic procedure had been performed, and

(6) to automate the fiscal functions of a clinical laboratory.

TESTING FOR APTITUDE

During the summer of 1965, every one of the fifty employees in the Central Laboratory, with one exception (a laboratory aide), took a written test for aptitude in data processing. Interestingly enough, the eight members of this group who demonstrated the greatest aptitude and interest were the supervisors of the major areas of the Central Laboratory. This group became the nucleus for the development of the laboratory system. Starting in December, 1964, and extending throughout 1965, this group learned a new language.

LANGUAGE OF THE COMPUTER

Our initial reaction to a data processing organization, its personnel, and equipment was one of bewilderment, awe, and envy. We saw eager, bright young men and attractive women of a single mode speaking precisely and authoritatively in a foreign language and working in a noiseless, air conditioned, and totally controlled environment in which stood rectangular boxes with lights which blinked incessantly. Most of us, accustomed to survival under stress and under less than ideal working conditions, reacted instinctively with fear and suspicion. And the computer experts, who were to us a new and separate breed, appeared to gloat in this mystique.

In order to communicate with these individuals, it was necessary to learn the language of the computer.[9] As we became better acquainted with the basic concepts of the computer, we recognized how inherently precise its logic is. Eventually we recognized that a computer is an electro-mechanical conglomerate which was built by engineers who understood the binary language of elec-

[9]Lord Bowden: The language of computers. *Am Scientist, 58:*43-53, 1970.

tricity. The computer is a big dumb brute. This realization gave us more confidence.

The language of the computer is elegant beyond any description in its spartan simplicity. Its alphabet consists of one and zero. The one represents an electrical pulse or bit and the zero represents no pulse or no bit. With just these two symbols, many different information codes can be developed.[10] The basic code in most computers is based on the binary number system. In a binary number, the first right hand column represents units and the value increases only twice each time one moves one place to the left. The two binary symbols can be coded to represent any number, alphabetic character, punctuation mark or special symbol. The reader is referred to other sources for a detailed discussion of the computer language.[11,12,13] Our purpose in mentioning it here is merely to stress that an understanding of the fundamentals of the computer language assists immeasurably in dispelling the fear and suspicion of the unknown demon.

TRAINING OF THE STAFF

The manufacturer supplied an instructor who lectured to the supervisors, beginning with basic computer concepts, the computer language and the hardware components. Programmed instruction material was supplied to us on communicating with the 1401 computer. By the summer of 1965, the group had progressed to mastery of the programmed instruction material concerning the Fortran language. A programmed instruction course in basic computer concepts and Fortran was offered during this time to all interested laboratory personnel. In November, 1965, the supervisors attended a course in 1130 Assembler language. By this time it was becoming evident that only a chosen few with certain innate talents and interests were endowed with the ability to converse

[10]*Basic Computer Systems Principles. Vol. 1, 2, 3.* Programmed Instruction Course. International Business Machines Corporation, 1964.

[11]E.M. Awad, and Data Processing Management Association: *Automatic Data Processing. Principles and Procedures.* Englewood Cliffs, Prentice-Hall, 1966.

[12]F. Stuart: *Introductory Computer Programming.* N.Y., Wiley & Sons, 1966.

[13]S.O. Krasnoff: *Computers in Medicine. A Primer for the Practicing Physician.* Springfield, Thomas, 1967.

fluently with the computer. By November, 1965, the supervisors had completed the formal program for learning the basic language of the computer and were ready for the next logical step—a systems analysis of the Central Laboratory.

SYSTEMS ANALYSIS

The term *systems analysis* evokes in the minds of the uninitiated an impression of some mysterious process whereby an expert makes the computer work. There is nothing magical about the process. It is the logical approach to problem-solving which is the stock-in-trade of the experimental scientist and which a clinician applies intuitively in his management of a patient. One first defines the problem by collecting data concerning all the variables involved and then outlines step by step the most efficient solution to this problem. In the process, since the computer is so logical, one must define in minute detail precisely each sequential step; otherwise the computer will not accept the solution. The proof of the solution of the problem, as far as the computer is concerned, is that the program written for the solution actually runs on the computer.

SYSTEMS ANALYSIS OF A CLINICAL LABORATORY

The primary responsibility of a clinical laboratory is to generate information in the form of numbers and descriptions with maximum efficiency, accuracy, and speed, and at least cost. This task commences with the proper procurement and identification of the biological specimen from the patient; the process continues with the actual performance of the analytical procedure, followed by the arithmetic calculations, and ends in a legible written report which is incorporated in the clinical record.

●●●●●●●●●●●●●●●●●●●●●●●●●●●●

CHAPTER IV

A COMPUTERIZED SYSTEM FOR THE CENTRAL LABORATORY

PLANS FOR IMPLEMENTATION

WEEKLY MEETINGS of the supervisors began in November, 1965, for the purpose of a systems analysis of the Central Laboratory. It was necessary to collect data concerning the number and types of analyses performed by each section, the temporal distribution of the workload and its sources, the nature of the information required for the financial record and the charging mechanism, and the time spent by the laboratory staff in the performance of each function.

Once systems analysis had defined the prerequisites of the system, the staff developed a detailed plan for the implementation of the data processing within our laboratory. We defined the minimal amount of information about the patient required to properly identify and process each specimen: name, age, sex, hospital number, location in the hospital, and indicators of financial status. The decision was made to put this information into the computer (to *input*) by means of a Hollerith-coded card; a card format was designed for this purpose. The results of the laboratory tests initially were to be inputted by means of an optical mark page reader (an IBM 1232). This meant then that a system had to be designed to identify each specimen within the laboratory by some numerical code, since it would be cumbersome to use the name of the patient. Once the information for the identification of the sample and the patient were inputted to the computer, files could be developed in the computer for storage of the information. The nature of the organization of the record in the computer file required considerable thought in order that the

19

information could be *massaged* in every conceivable manner. The information then must be *outputted* by some means. The method selected was to use a line printer for chart reports and typewriters for communication within the laboratory.

During this period in early 1966 the question was first raised as to whether the laboratory should introduce a screening battery of biochemical tests. A decision was made to design the system so that each AutoAnalyzer could be considered by the computer as a discrete process controlled unit. The backup for the system was to be the usual visual one, the traditional strip chart of the recorder. A computer program would be developed to monitor the analog signal, to identify each peak at maximum height, to scrutinize its configuration for validity, and to store this information and to compare the value with those of the standards, to calculate the algebraic values, and to merge this information with the data that identified the sample and patient.

By early January, 1966, it was possible to flow-chart the overall system. Each specimen was to be assigned a sequential four-digit number; a separate request card was designed for each individual test. The analyses would be performed on the AutoAnalyzer or manually and the results would be written on the card. The card would then be keypunched with this information and inputted to the system by means of the card reader. Further efforts then were devoted to development of the format of the records on disk.

FUNCTIONAL COMPONENTS OF THE 1800 PROCESS CONTROL MONITOR

The IBM 1800 laboratory instruments monitoring system provided for an initial capability of monitoring thirty-two low-level signals. The signals from the instruments go to the analog-to-digital converter (ADC). The ADC converts the analog signal to a digital value (Fig. 3).

The digitized signal next enters the 1802-I central processor. The central processing unit contains main core memory for storage of programs and data during processing and the arithmetic/logic circuits which process calculations and logic operations. The characteristics of the 1802-I were as follows: 16K, 4 microsecond

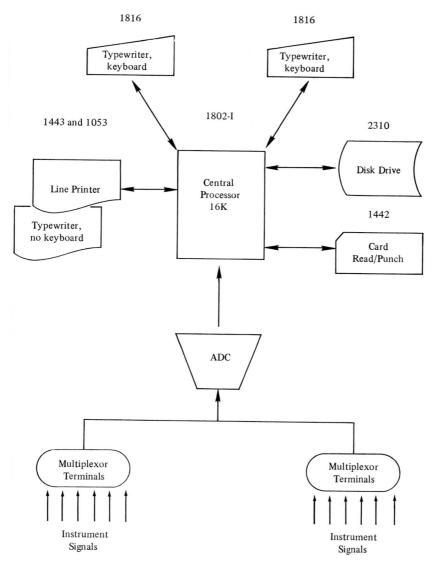

Figure 3. The functional components of the process control monitoring system of the Central Laboratory.

memory; 16 bit, binary word, plus a parity bit and a storage protect bit; three index registers; twelve levels of priority interrupts; four data channels; three interval timers; console; and a magnetic tape input/output (I/O) control.

After processing, the data may be stored in the 2310 *disk drive* which provides for storage of over a million characters of data on-line.

The 1442 *card read/punch* provides a card reading and punching facility. The functions of this equipment are program loading, data entry, and record punching. Cards can be inputted at the rate of three hundred per minute and outputted at sixty per minute.

The two 1816 *typewriters* provided two discrete locations for the entry of alphanumeric information and for systems inquiry.

The 1443 *line printer* and 1053 *typewriter without keyboard* were to be used for output of information from the system. The 1053 printed at the rate of fifteen characters per second, while the 1443 printed 120 lines per minute.

The initial cost of this system was $1,954.00/month on a rental basis or $83,722.00 for outright purchase. The institution chose to rent. The system was originally scheduled for delivery in mid-February, 1966.

APPOINTMENT OF A LABORATORY COMPUTER SYSTEMS DESIGNER

In June, 1966, the junior author, who was previously the supervisor in the Clinical Microbiology section, was appointed Laboratory Computer Systems Designer. He left for San Jose and San Francisco to gain *hands-on* experience on the 1800 system. Another supervisor was assigned full-time to the programming of the system. In the meantime, detailed physical plans for the installation of the system were initiated. The requirements for electrical power, temperature and humidity control, proper spacing of the hardware, accessibility of the computer room to the laboratory, provisions for false flooring, all were subjects discussed in considerable detail.

OTHER 1800 LABORATORY SYSTEMS

During the fall of 1966, the Director of Laboratory Services visited other laboratories with similar plans for automation and computerization. The Kings County Research Laboratory in Brooklyn, New York, already had several lines of AutoAnalyzers which were monitored by an 1800 process control computer. This system had been designed to *batch process* large numbers of samples in a private commercial laboratory. An elaborate software program had been developed to analyze the analog signals (the peak-picking routine) and to correct for baseline drift and sample interaction, but none of it was available even to an educational institution. And so it was necessary to re-invent the wheel. The Johns Hopkins Hospital's 1800 on-line system which was designed primarily for chemical analysis, was just being *de-bugged*. Dr. William R. Robinson, III, at the Bowman Gray School of Medicine had succeeded in coupling AutoAnalyzers to the 1800 and had written his own *peak-picking routine,* which he generously offered to share with us; this program was received in January, 1966.

The 1800 system was originally scheduled for delivery in September, 1966. This was about the time that we were introduced to a new terminology in computer marketing—*slippage.* Slippage is an unavoidable delay in the delivery schedule which is most probably due to an overzealous marketing staff promising customers too much too soon. The delivery date of the 1800 *slipped* to February, 1967, and then subsequently to June, 1967.

DEVELOPMENT OF THE DATA PROCESSING ROUTINES

In the meantime, in November, 1966, the planning group of supervisors started to program the data processing routines. The routines were ready for testing by March of 1967, when news was received of the delay in the delivery of the 1800. In desperation, an 1130 computer was rented for the testing because the 1130 has data processing capability identical to that of the 1800 but without the process control features. Initially, therefore, our efforts were devoted to perfecting the data processing system. On April

15, 1967, the optical mark page reader was delivered. In our original plan, we intended to develop printed $8\frac{1}{2}'' \times 11''$ scan sheets which contained all necessary identifying information required for the technologist to report the results of analyses.

On May 5, 1967, the 1800 system was finally delivered; the

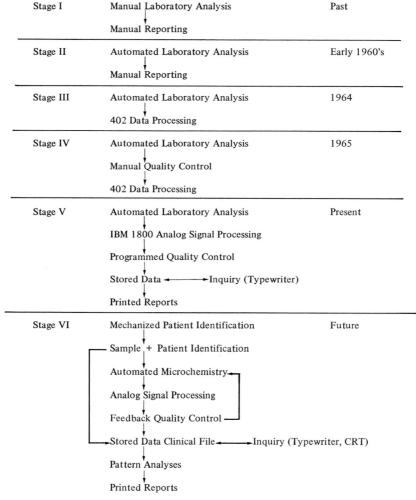

Figure 4. The evolution of an automated computerized system for a clinical laboratory.

elapsed time between initial proposal and planning and delivery was twenty-five months. During the period from July, 1967, through November, 1967, many attempts were made to implement the use of the optical mark page reader as the primary input device. Because of poor systems design, all efforts were unsuccessful. Our staff found that entry of numerical information by this method was too tedious and that the error rate in transcription averaged 20 percent even in the hands of interested participants. Further, parallel runs of inputting information by means of hand written results which were subsequently keypunched versus inputting identical information through the optical mark page reader revealed that the latter was slower and more prone to error. We reluctantly were forced to the conclusion that the optical mark page reader was unsuitable for this laboratory.

By Thanksgiving of 1967, we realized that the amount of data being generated in the Clinical Chemistry laboratory was too great to be handled by an off-line data processing system. The solution appeared to be the obvious one of reducing the data handling by coupling the AutoAnalyzers directly to the 1800. After many months of struggling to mimic the 402 system for the 1800, we awoke to the fact that we were not using the 1800 for the purpose for which it was originally designed.

●●●●●●●●●●●●●●●●●●●●●●●●●●●●

CHAPTER V

THE PROCESS CONTROL MONITORING SYSTEM FOR CLINICAL CHEMISTRY

DEVELOPMENT OF THE AUTOANALYZER MONITORING SYSTEM

MOST OF THE early planning efforts had been devoted to development of the data processing system off-line. We had overlooked the fundamental fact that the 1800 computer had been designed primarily as a process control monitor. On December 27, 1967, the decision was made to place the glucose channel of Auto-Analyzer on-line to the 1800 as soon as possible. This meant that it was necessary for us to develop a *standard operating procedure*. After much discussion it was decided that whenever a technologist began analysis on any channel, the first eight of the forty positions on the turntable would be reserved for increasing concentrations of standards. Initially, positions 9, 10, and 11 were reserved for standards to be used to correct for sample interaction. Positions 12, 13, and 14 were reserved for quality control specimens. Two of the three quality control specimens were to be within ± 2 standard deviations of the respective mean values; otherwise, the system was programmed to reject additional signals. It was the responsibility of the technologist to trouble shoot and to correct the problems and to restart the run. The system, therefore, was designed to give maximum responsibility to the staff for its management.

In an automated flow system of chemical analysis, sample interaction is said to be a problem affecting precision.[14] Data obtained under actual working conditions in our laboratory revealed that

---

[14]M.A. Evenson, Hicks, G.P., and Thiers, R.E.: Peak characteristics and computers in continuous flow analysis. *Clin Chem, 16*:606-611, 1970.

26

this interaction averaged about 5 percent for the following determinations: glucose, urea, creatinine, calcium and protein-bound iodine. Since 5 percent was considerably less than the average reproducibility by the manual methods, the decision was made to simplify the programming by disregarding this factor.

PEAK-PICKING ROUTINE

The electrical signal from the colorimeter circuit in an Auto-Analyzer is an analog voltage which varies between 0 and 50 millivolts and typically rises abruptly from a baseline to a peak and subsides to near baseline before rising again. In order to provide the computer with an analog signal of sufficient voltage, each AutoAnalyzer was modified by attaching a potentiometer to the slide-wire drive gear. A constant 5-volt DC power supply was connected across this potentiometer. The wiper and common terminals were connected to the analog input terminals of the 1800.

Although nominally designed to perform analyses regularly at forty to sixty per hour, the timing is dependent upon mechanical cams and is not consistent enough to monitor with an internal clock in the computer. The decision was made in November, 1967, to develop a unique system for coupling the AutoAnalyzer to the 1800 computer. Although we had access to the Fortran program for peak-picking from the Bowman Gray School of Medicine, this comprehensive program was too large, unfortunately, to fit into the 16K of core memory in our 1800. Mr. Pinfield, therefore, designed a simplified routine in Assembler language. This core limitation forced us also to design a hardware process interrupt.

DEVELOPMENT OF A HARDWARE PROCESS INTERRUPT

In retrospect, it is amusing and satisfying to recall that IBM with all its resources was incapable or unwilling to assist us in solving this problem of a hardware process interrupt and slope detector. A physician, a medical technologist with a hobby of electronics, and a graduate student in electrical engineering solved the problem. They developed an analog slope detector which notified the computer by means of an interrupt signal whenever a peak started. This device has an adjustable sensitivity to provide for variations in the roughness of each baseline; it could be so regulated that no signal would be given unless a true peak was detected. The start of the first peak causes the baseline reading to be stored and a program indicator to be set so that the analog input is scanned for the high point within the time interval expected for each peak. When the top of the peak is detected, the value is stored in core. At intervals of six minutes, this core table is written on the disk and cleared, and the calculation routine is initiated.

When the technologist enters the start code of an analyzer, a program is executed which sets to zero the appropriate temporary tables for peaks and results, resets indexes, and sets program indicators to show which channels have been started. The peak-picking routine is initiated and the computer begins scanning the analog input every two seconds.

IDENTIFICATION OF ANALYZER CHANNEL TO THE COMPUTER

An area on one of the disk files is reserved for information from each AutoAnalyzer channel. In this file are stored the number and concentration of the standards, limits for the control sera, turntable speed (indicating the expected duration of the peak for each sample) and information concerning whether or not the test requires a blank. An area is also reserved for temporary storage of peak values and results.

Each analyzer is assigned a number, and another disk file defines the channels which are associated with each analyzer. If the analyzer performs more than one type of test on the same channel, each test is assigned a number and treated as if it were a separate channel.

All programs pertaining to the collection of data from the on-line AutoAnalyzers are initiated from the laboratory by entering the analyzer number and program code number through the digital input terminals.

STRUCTURE OF THE FILE ON DISK

Since 40 percent of our work is for the Outpatient Department and since only one or two samples per outpatient are submitted each week, we organize our files by sample rather than by patient. This plan also permits us to process samples before detailed information about the patient is entered. Another consideration is that many readings fall outside the range permitted by the method, and in such cases the analysis has to be repeated on a diluted sample. Our system allows the technologist to analyze both a diluted and undiluted sample in the same run when there is reason to suspect that the results of the undiluted sample might be out of range.

LABORATORY TERMINALS

The system requires that the technologist inform the computer of both the access number and the location on the turntable of a particular specimen (Fig. 5). Here again IBM offered very little assistance in solving the problem as inexpensively as possible. To be sure, matrix keyboards were available but we could not afford them. Our engineer constructed a digital-input device (twelve rotary switches with settings 0-9) to allow input of data and control of program from the laboratory; the cost for each was about $600 (Fig. 6). A typewriter (for output only) was placed beside each of these digital input devices. Thus a means was established for communicating with the computer and for receiving messages.

An embryonic on-line, real-time, computerized data processing system finally became operational in October, 1968. It has been in continuous operation since then with a minimum amount of downtime.

OPERATION OF THE SYSTEM IN THE LABORATORY

Samples received in the laboratory are accompanied by multiple copy request forms (Fig. 5). Each sample is assigned a four digit laboratory accession number, which is attached to the sample and to the request form and is also entered in the log book. The sample is centrifuged, split, and distributed to the area (s) within

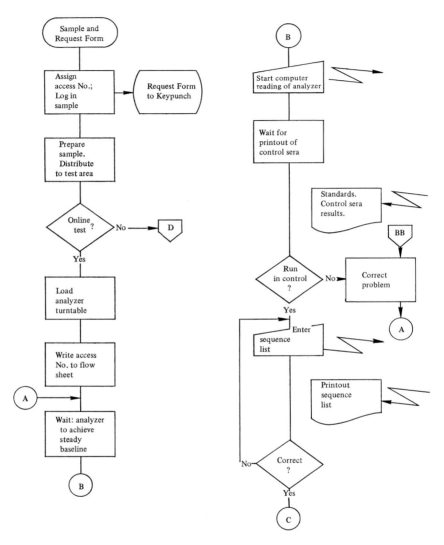

Figure 5. A flowchart of the operation of the Clinical Chemistry system.

the laboratory where the work will be performed. One copy of the request form is forwarded to the computer area, where a name card containing the accession number, identification of the pa-

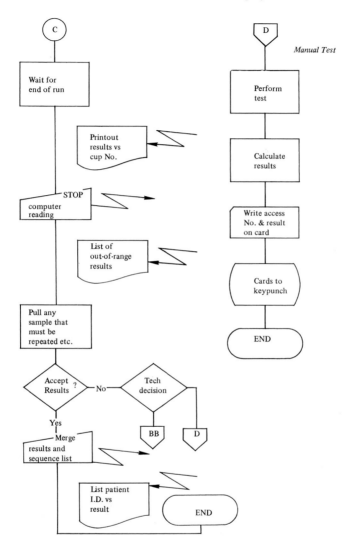

tient (name, hospital number, and location within the hospital),
and the type of specimen is keypunched.

Tests not carried out by an on-line AutoAnalyzer are performed and calculated manually, and the results are reported by

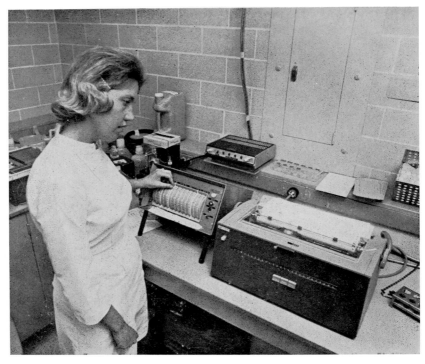

Figure 6. The digital-input device to allow input of data and control of program from the laboratory is located to the left of the output typewriter.

writing the sample accession number and the results onto a prepunched test card. A different card is required for each test.

On-line tests are performed as follows: The technologist loads the AutoAnalyzer turntable with standards and three control sera according to the standard operating procedure for the analysis being performed. Next, sample from patients are loaded onto the turntable. As the samples are poured into the cups, the turntable cup number, the accession number, and the dilution factor are written on the flow sheet. After every eight to ten samples, the *blank* cup is filled with water. After the analyzer has achieved a steady baseline state, the technologist initiates the run by turning on the sampler and signaling the computer to start reading the analog signal for this analyzer. In order to insure optimal accuracy and rapid reporting of results, only twenty-five to thirty unknowns are included in each run, although a larger number of unknowns can be analyzed at the discretion of the technologist.

After the peaks for the standards and control sera have been read, the computer calculates the values for the control sera from the standard curve and compares the results with limits stored in the disk file. Peak readings for the standard and results for the controls are typed on the typewriter in the laboratory (Fig. 7). If

```
START OF GLUC ANALYZER   22.10

LINE  1  GLUCOSE                    3.30    22.30

STANDARDS
CONC          0.0     50.0   100.0    150.0    200.0      250.0     300.0
READING    3400.0   4696.0 6872.0  10488.0  16552.0    25160.0  29976.0
   2 SD  LIMITS    46.2  TO    52.1  LOW   CONTROL =     51.8
   2 SD  LIMITS    97.0  TO   106.1  MED   CONTROL =    100.2
   2 SD  LIMITS   190.1  TO   207.3  HIGH  CONTROL =    196.0
RUN IN CONTROL
CUP NO.       12      13      14      15      16      17
RESULT      81.7  9999.0   -1.0   100.2   101.1    82.8


          LINE  1  GLUCOSE               3.30    22.36
CUP NO.       18      19      20      21      22      23
RESULT      63.9    95.9    -1.0    -1.0    -1.0    -1.0


          LINE  1  GLUCOSE               3.30    22.42
CUP NO.       24      25      26      27
RESULT     120.0    85.1    -1.0    -1.0
```

Figure 7. Sample of lab printout for an on-line run of glucose.
Explanation
Result 9999 = Reading above high standard
Result −1 = No peak detected

The glucose analyzer was started at 22.10 hours on March 30. Twenty minutes after the start, peaks for standards and controls had been read. Values for control sera were calculated and compared to the stored ranges; they were found to be within acceptable limits and the computer accepted the run as being in control.

Note that the reading for cup 13 was greater than the high standard, and that this *high* swamped the peak for the following sample. The technologist recognized this problem, diluted the high sample, and placed the dilution at the end of the run. The swamped sample was also repeated.

Every six minutes results were calculated and printed by the computer. The −1 results here are readings obtained from water samples.

```
ENTER GLUC SEQUENCE LIST
    12   1736      DOE, JANE          123456      0       0
    13   1737      SMITH, BILL        234567      0       0
    14   1743      BROWN, JOHN        345678      0       0
    15   1744      DOE, JOHN          246802      0       0
    16   1750      JONES, JOHN        390242      0       0
    17   1755      GREEN, MARY        357913      0       0
    18   1758      BLUE, FRED         135791      0       0
    19   1763      OTHER, A.N.        111222      0       0
    20    10       CONTROL/H20
    21    10       CONTROL/H20
    22    10       CONTROL/H20
    23    10       CONTROL/H20
    24   1737      SMITH, BILL        234567      3       2
    25   1743      BROWN, JOHN        345678      0       2


         STOP   OF GLUC ANALYZER   22.50
         GLUC  CHECK LIST
         CUP  ACCNO      GLUC
          13   1737      9999
          14   1743        -1
         END OF CHECK LIST


DO NOT START GLUC ANALYZER UNTIL NEXT MESSAGE
MOVE AND LIST RESULTS   23.00
    CUP  ACCNO                             GLUC
      8     1      CONTROL/H20              52
      9     2      CONTROL/H20             100
     10     3      CONTROL/H20             196
     12   1736     DOE, JANE                82
     13   1737     SMITH, BILL            9999
     14   1743     BROWN, JOHN              -1
     15   1744     DOE, JOHN               100
     16   1750     JONES, JOHN             101
     17   1755     GREEN, MARY              83
     18   1758     BLUE, FRED               64
     19   1763     OTHER A,N                96
     20    10      CONTROL/H20              -1
     21    10      CONTROL/H20              -1
     22    10      CONTROL/H20              -1
     23    10      CONTROL/H20              -1
     24   1737     SMITH, BILL   x  3   OLAY   360
     25   1743     BROWN, JOHN           OLAY    85
YOU MAY NOW START GLUC ANALYZER
```

Figure 8. Samples of laboratory printout of the sequence list, check list, and the merged file containing the identifying information and the results.
Explanation

    The technologist entered the sequence of samples and for cups 24 and

two or more of the controls are out of limits, the computer stops reading that analyzer and types a message in the laboratory that the run has been aborted. If the run is accepted, the computer will calculate results for the unknowns every six minutes, store them on disk, and type the cup numbers and corresponding numbers on the typewriter in the laboratory.

While the run is in progress, the technologist sends to the computer, by means of the digital input device, the sequence of samples that was written down earlier on the flowsheet. She enters the turntable cup number, the accession number, the dilution factor, and a code if this sample is being repeated. There are two options for the repeat code: A code of *1* will overlay the results of the current test on all previous results; a code of *2* will overlay the results of the current test only on results which were previously out of range. The second repeat code allows the sample to be run undiluted and diluted in the same batch, and the program will save the results of the least dilute sample for which the result is in range. Analysis of a sample can be repeated as often as necessary to obtain a valid result (Fig. 8) .

When the run is complete, the technologist signals the computer that the analyzer has stopped. This signal automatically executes a program to type a list of out-of-range peaks, indicating which samples must be analyzed again (Fig. 8) . If any peaks were detected on blank samples, this fact will be printed as a warning that the sequence list is incorrect or that there is a problem with the computer reading of the run.

---

25 entered the code of 2 to indicate repeats. A 3 was also entered for cup 24 to indicate a three-fold dilution.

The analyzer was stopped at 22.50 hours and the two out-of-range results were printed out.

The upper sequence list is typed out after the technologist has inputted the routine to merge the Sequence list with the results and to transfer the merged data to the permanent files. The listing indicated that the sample in cup 24 was diluted three-fold. The printed result has been adjusted by the factor. The results printed for cups 24 and 25 have replaced (overlaid) previous results, in this case those for cups 13 and 14. If the high sample had not been diluted in time for this run, it could have been placed in a subsequent run with the proper repeat code and dilution factor; the same overlaying process would have taken place.

It remains the technologist's responsibility to verify the accuracy of the results. When she is satisfied that they are correct, she initiates another program to merge the sequence list and the results. This program also transfers the data to another file, from which a preliminary report can be printed. If a repeat code was entered, results which were previously out-of-limit are deleted. Finally, the program types a list of the patient's names and the results of their tests for laboratory records (Fig. 8). Once results have been transferred to the print files, they can be retrieved at any time by entering the accession number and initiating the *inquiry* program from a disk to input terminal. Accession numbers can be found by referring to the laboratory log book or the alphabetic listing of patients' names and accession numbers (Fig. 9). This listing is updated daily.

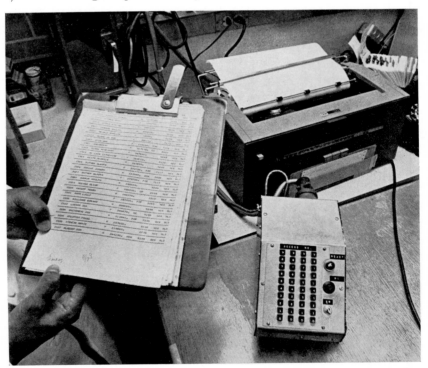

Figure 9. The inquiry terminal for retrieval of information by accession number.

OPERATION IN THE COMPUTER ROOM

As frequently as is convenient, name cards and result cards are keypunched and fed into the computer to be written onto disk files. Twice each day, all available results are sorted by sample and *chart copy* reports are printed. Carbon copies of these reports are kept on file in the laboratory. Preliminary results are printed and distributed as soon as possible after the completion of a run. Because of limitation of disk space, results are kept available for on-line inquiry for ten days only. At the end of this time, the data are transferred to magnetic tape for permanent storage.

CHAPTER VI

THE DATA PROCESSING SYSTEM FOR CLINICAL MICROBIOLOGY

BACKGROUND

CURRENT METHODS for the identification of most micro-organisms require that these organisms which are resident in the biologic specimens be given an opportunity to grow in or on selected media. A considerable amount of art is involved in the decision-making steps required to identify a specific micro-organism. This analytic process requires intuition, experience, and serendipity and cannot be defined with total objectivity at the present time. The aura of mysticism and of craftsmanship still pervades microbiology. A possible new approach for more rapid and specific identification would be the application of tagged immunologic reagents, such as specific antibodies, but such attempts are still in the experimental stage. Thus, the actual laboratory procedures for the isolation and the identification of micro-organisms and their testing for sensitivity to various antibiotics are not yet amenable to automation and computerization.

The data processing, however, can be computerized, provided the staff in the microbiology laboratory would compromise upon a standard scheme for identification of micro-organisms and a standard nomenclature for description of their findings. Agreement among the staff members upon these points would be by itself a major accomplishment.

SYSTEMS DESIGN

During the period in which the clinical chemistry system was evolving, a separate task force was formed in August, 1968, to develop a unique data processing system for clinical microbiology. An assistant supervisor spent four months in the systems design;

an instructor, a month in the development of the computer file. One programmer spent a year on the project. During February and March of 1969 the entire staff participated in the documentation of the actual data processing requirements in the laboratory. Following this, the requirements of a master file were defined. Agreement was reached among the staff upon a standard nomenclature for organisms and a common language for other descriptors. A total of 1,250 codes sufficed to identify all organisms and to provide the additional text material needed to describe all findings. The decision was made originally in April, 1969, to input data via a document reader, but this plan was subsequently abandoned because of difficulty in communicating with the one manufacturer who had the desirable hardware. There was no alternative but to design a system to input all data in coded form via cards that were keypunched by an operator.

THE ORIGINAL SYSTEM

After additional programming and trial runs, the original system became operational on July 20, 1970, after almost two years of planning. All information from the Clinical Microbiology laboratory was successfully entered into a computer file using keypunched cards as input, and printed reports were available for distribution by 2 p.m. daily. The technologists discovered that the standardized data processing system required slightly more of their time but that the advantages of a printed report and the retrieval capabilities of the system far outweighed this one disadvantage.

Because the system required at least four hours of keypunching time each day, we began re-exploring the use of a document reader for input of information. It required an additional two years of planning and negotiation before we were able, on June 29, 1972, to convert completely to an optical scanner interfaced to a keypunch for producing the primary input for Clinical Microbiology. It was immediately evident that this device was far superior to manual keypunching.

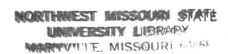

DESCRIPTION OF THE CURRENT SYSTEM

The *objectives* of this data processing system are to collect and store data from the Clinical Microbiology laboratory in order to provide multiple copies of printed reports, to generate charges automatically, and to provide for on-line inquiry for results on the most recent samples and an efficient method for retrieving data which have been stored for a longer period.

Our approach is to keep data on disk files until all work on a sample is completed and for a reasonable time thereafter in order to permit on-line inquiry for these results. Since there is a considerable difference in the time required to complete work on samples depending upon the type of culture or test requested, the samples are divided into three groups:

1. cultures for acid fast bacilli and fungi; information is kept on disk for 10 weeks.
2. blood cultures; kept on disk for 4 weeks.
3. routine cultures and serology; kept for 3 weeks.

Data for each group of samples are kept on a separate disk file and each group is referenced by its own accession number series.

To store results in the computer, we assign a code number to the name of each organism, the sample source, the comment and the growth evaluation. These code numbers refer to a file of English language statements from which the printed report is formatted.

The *input document* is the machine readable sheet marked by the technologist during the analysis. One of the six sheets in use is shown in Figure 10. Whenever possible this sheet is designed in such a way that the technologist places one mark to identify both the organism and the degree of growth. When an unusual organism is recovered, the technologist is required to enter its code number on the sheet.

OPERATION OF THE SYSTEM IN THE LABORATORY

A specimen is received, accompanied by a multiple part request form (Fig. 11). The technologist assigns to this specimen the next accession number from the appropriate series. She affixes a label, preprinted with this number, to the request form, as well

RESPIRATORY—GENITAL—MISCELLANEOUS—BLOOD

ACCESSION NUMBER											
		0	1	2	3	4	5	6	7	8	9
		0	1	2	3	4	5	6	7	8	9
		0	1	2	3	4	5	6	7	8	9
		0	1	2	3	4	5	6	7	8	9
		RESP 0		GENIT 3		MISC 5		BLOOD 9			

		RESP	GENIT	MISC	BLOOD		
NO GROWTH IN DAYS		0	1	2			
		0	1	2	3	4	5	6	7	8	9

Organism	Code	RESP	GENIT	MISC	BLOOD
STAPHYLOCOCCUS AUREUS	(0414)	11	1	3	5	7	9
STAPHYLOCOCCUS EPIDERMIDIS	(0415)	11	1	3	5	7	9
DIPLOCOCCUS PNEUMONIAE	(041C)	11	1	3	5	7	9
STREPTOCOCCUS PYOGENES, GROUP A	(0421)	11	1	3	5	7	9
STREPTOCOCCUS, BETA HEM NOT GROUP A	(0417)	11	1	3	5	7	9
STREPTOCOCCUS, BETA HEM NOT GROUP A OR D	(0418)	11	1	3	5	7	9
STREPTOCOCCUS, GROUP D (ENTEROCOCCUS)	(0419)	11	1	3	5	7	9
STREPTOCOCCUS VIRIDANS GROUP	(0422)	11	1	3	5	7	9
STREPTOCOCCUS, NONHEMOLYTIC	(0420)	11	1	3	5	7	9
NEISSERIA	(0318)	11	1	3	5	7	9
MICROCOCCUS	(0413)	11	1	3	5	7	9
DIPHTHEROIDS	(0409)	11	1	3	5	7	9
LACTOBACILLUS	(0411)	11	1	3	5	7	9
CANDIDA ALBICANS	(0557)	11	1	3	5	7	9
YEAST	(0553)	11	1	3	5	7	9
HEMOPHILUS	(0313)	11	1	3	5	7	9
GRAM—RODS	(0811)	11	1	3	5	7	9
E. COLI	(0153)	11	1	3	5	7	9
KLEBSIELLA	(0167)	11	1	3	5	7	9
ENTEROBACTER	(0158)	11	1	3	5	7	9
PROTEUS MIRABILIS	(0175)	11	1	3	5	7	9
PSEUDOMONAS AERUGINOSA	(0324)	11	1	3	5	7	9
BACTEROIDES	(0505)	11	1	3	5	7	9
HERELLEA	(0314)	11	1	3	5	7	9
ENTEROBACTER-KLEBSIELLA GROUP	(0162)	11	1	3	5	7	9
PROTEUS SP.	(0174)	11	1	3	5	7	9
C. VAGINALIS	(1095)	11	1	3	5	7	9

OTHER: (__ __ __ __)
- 0 1 2
- 9 1 2 3 4 5 6 7 8 9
- 0 1 2 3 4 5 6 7 8 9
- 0 1 2 3 4 5 6 7 8 9
- WT. 11 1 3 5 7 9

OTHER: (__ __ __ __)
- 0 1 2
- 0 1 2 3 4 5 6 7 8 9
- 0 1 2 3 4 5 6 7 8 9
- 0 1 2 3 4 5 6 7 8 9
- WT. 11 1 3 5 7 9

OTHER: (__ __ __ __)
- 0 1 2
- 0 1 2 3 4 5 6 7 8 9
- 0 1 2 3 4 5 6 7 8 9
- 0 1 2 3 4 5 6 7 8 9
- WT. 11 1 3 5 7 9

NO BETA STREP GROWN	(0855)	11	
CULTURE NOT STREAKED FOR ISOLATION	(0881)	11	PLEASE REPEAT (0791) 9
SPECIMEN RECEIVED ON SWAB	(0841)	11	
THIO BROTH ONLY INOCULATED	(0837)	11	
NO NEISSERIA GONORRHEAE GROWN	(0856)	11	WRONG OR INADEQUATE
SPECIMEN NOT INOCULATED ANAEROBICALLY	(0844)	11	MEDIA INOC. (0790) 9
NO GROWTH ON PLATES IN 2 DAYS	(0874)	11	
DOCTOR NOTIFIED BY PHONE	(0873)	11	
SEE PREVIOUS CULTURE FOR SENSITIVITIES	(0904)	11	
SUPPLEMENTARY REPORT	(0871)	11	

TECH. I.D.   PEDS 11   0 1 2 3 4 5 6 7 8 9

CONTROL NUMBER

Bell&Howell 7812-022

Figure 10. An example of the input document in the Clinical Microbiology laboratory.

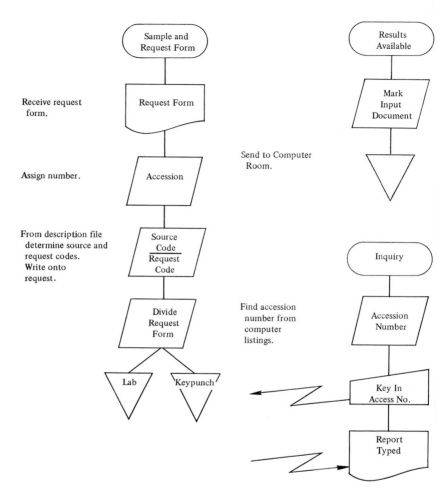

Figure 11. A flowchart of the data processing routines in the Clinical Microbiology laboratory.

as to the specimen, the media to which it will be inoculated, and the appropriate input document. In addition, the technologist writes onto the request form the source code number which describes the specimen and the request code number which identifies the charge, for example, 53-106 (vaginal-GC screening) or

34-106 (serum-ASO titer). A copy of the request form is then sent to the computer room.

As results are available, the technologist marks the input document. These forms are collected periodically and sent to the computer room where they are scanned with the document reader and the data are keypunched automatically for input to the computer files.

On-line inquiry for results is processed as follows: The accession number for the sample is obtained from the listings printed by computer. This number is keyed into the inquiry terminal in the laboratory. The computer then searches the disk files and types back a report.

OPERATION IN THE COMPUTER ROOM

Patient identification is generated by keypunching a name card for each sample (Fig. 12). Each name card contains the following information: The name, age, sex, hospital number and nursing unit number of the patient; the date and time of receipt of the specimen, its accession number, and its source and test request code numbers.

The *results* of the microbiological studies are read by the document reader from the input document and keypunched into cards. This information is then inputted via the card reader as soon as possible in order to keep the information in the disk files current.

Once daily, *reports* that contain all results entered during the previous twenty-four hours are printed for each sample.

Cards which contain the patient's hospital number and the codes indicating the *charges* are generated daily for the main hospital computer system.

In the daily file maintenance routines, current *listings of samples* by patient name and by accession number are printed for the laboratory, and the oldest data are purged from the disk files and stored on magnetic tape. These tape files are our permanent record and are used for retrieval of old results and for generation of *statistical reports* such as a monthly summary of the workload and of patterns of antibiotic sensitivity for each organism.

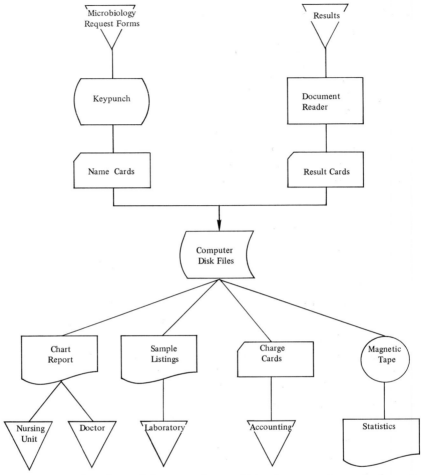

Figure 12. A flowchart of the procedures within the computer room for processing data from the Clinical Microbiology laboratory.

FUTURE PLANS

We plan next to acquire a document reader for installation within the Clinical Microbiology laboratory so that results can be inputted on-line to the computer as soon as the work is completed. Routines will be written to verify the information before it is stored in a permanent file.

A system has been evolved for the data processing requirements of a clinical microbiology laboratory.

CHAPTER VII

THE DATA PROCESSING SYSTEM
FOR HEMATOLOGY

I N SEPTEMBER, 1968, prior to the time that the clinical chemistry
system went on-line, work was already under way in the Hematology section on the design of forms for the input of laboratory
data via an optical mark page reader. The IBM 1232 system was
a failure in Clinical Chemistry and we learned that the most
efficient way to input data into the computer is directly on-line.

SYSTEMS ANALYSIS

Systems analysis of the work in the Hematology section revealed that approximately one-half of the total workload results in
numbers, such as the total red cell count, the total white cell
count, hemoglobin concentration, and prothrombin time. The
remaining one-half consists of descriptive information, such as
that concerning the blood smear and the urinary sediment. It
appeared very probable that the automated instruments already
in use or under development for this laboratory would have computer interfaces that were commercially available in the forseeable
future; therefore, the initial effort was directed towards the development of a special device to input into the 1800 the descriptive information derived from the examination of the peripheral
blood smear. Planning for this began in late September, 1968.

DEVELOPMENT OF HOTC

A terminal [HOTC (Hematology On-line To Computer)]
was designed for direct entry of the differential count and evaluation of the blood smear into the computer (Fig. 13). The differential count is performed on eight pushbutton switches which are
mounted on a small box; this count registers on an array of elec-

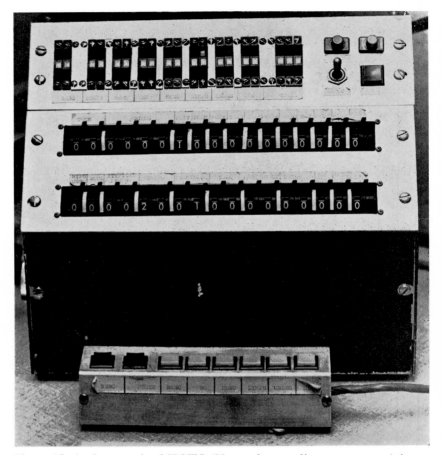

Figure 13. A photograph of HOTC (Hematology on-line to computer) input terminal.

tromechanical counters on the panel of the HOTC box. There are eight two-digit counters. Any count registering on counters 2-8 will also register on the three-digit *Total* counter. When the *Total* count reaches 100, a whistle blows and the counters are prevented from operating. Depressing the *Reset* switch resets all the counters to zero.

Data concerning identification and evaluation of cells are set on an array of thirty-four lever-operated rotary switches. Switches with two, five, and ten positions are provided for the various types of data. The *Platelet* switch is marked A-I-D for Average-Increase-Decrease.

A *Ready* light on the panel will be on if the computer is ready to accept data. When the differential count has been completed and the switches set, pressing the *Send* button will alert the computer.

The computer can read all the information from the panel, sixteen *bits* at a time, in eleven groups. If information is entered which is inconsistent or invalid from the standpoint of arithmetic or physiology, the computer will light the *Tilt* lamp.

A prototype of HOTC was available for testing by December, 1968. Preliminary trials in the routine laboratory raised some questions about the efficiency of this mode of data input. We have not yet decided that the input of the information from the peripheral smear via HOTC is ideal. If so, we will have to build several more of these special input devices. Moreover, we will need additional typewriters in order to verify the information being inputted via HOTC. Pending this decision, we have been developing a hard copy backup system which will use a document reader similar to that in the Clinical Microbiology system. Implementation of this system awaits acquisition of the hardware and the availability of funding for additional clerical personnel.

AUTOMATION IN HEMATOLOGY

A decision was made on April 17, 1969, to acquire the Coulter Model S particle counter. This instrument counts red cells and white cells in blood, determines hemoglobin concentration, and calculates the hematocrit and red cell indices; it prints values for these seven tests directly onto a report form within a matter of less than a minute from the time the specimen is introduced into the system. This single machine is capable of handling approximately one-half of the total workload in our Hematology laboratory.

Our emphasis shifted to interfacing the Coulter S to the 1800 because of the workload capability of the instrument as well as the fact that an interface had not been marketed. Completion of this project was delayed until October, 1970, because of the hardware constraints of the 1800 systems. That is to say, in 1969 we did not have adequate space on disk for storage of the information from the Hematology laboratory nor did we have the typewriter for communicating from the laboratory to the computer. At the present time the Coulter S interface to the 1800 is operational in conjunction with typewriter output concerned with the quality control program in the laboratory.

FUTURE PLANS

We are awaiting the acquisition of additional document readers to input the remaining information from the Hematology laboratory into the computer. Unless all information can be inputted, we would be faced with the poor economics of a dual system.

CHAPTER VIII

THE EVOLUTION OF THE HARDWARE

AN ADMONITION

IT IS WELL FOR ANYONE who is planning to deal with computer manufacturers to remember that in our capitalistic society the primary motive of private enterprise is profit. This being the case, the interface between the computer manufacturer and the medical user is oftentimes incompatible or at least bothersome. We have learned from experience to be wary of any claims for functional capabilities or promises of delivery dates for hardware. Yet, on the other hand, it is impossible to develop the system without the assistance of the computer manufacturer.

ADAPTATION TO NEED

The Central Laboratory 1800 system grew in a modular fashion with periodic upgrading of the hardware as the need arose. Keypunching has been the primary mode of data input since 1965 when we begun with the 402 accounting machine (Table I). The 402 system was removed in the fall of 1968. A 1232 optical mark page system for input was tried with unsuccessful results during 1967 and 1968.

UPGRADING OF THE CENTRAL PROCESSING UNIT

When the 1800 system was delivered in May, 1967, the central processor contained a core memory of 16,000 words (16K). Before we were even able to store data on magnetic tape, it was necessary in 1968 to improve the functional capabilities of this 16K of core memory. The core memory size was increased to 32K in 1969 in order to support data collection from additional lines of AutoAnalyzers. Soon thereafter, in early 1970, core speed was increased from four to two microseconds in order to accommo-

Table I

THE TEMPORAL RELATIONSHIPS OF CHANGES IN HARDWARE WITH FUNCTIONAL CHANGES

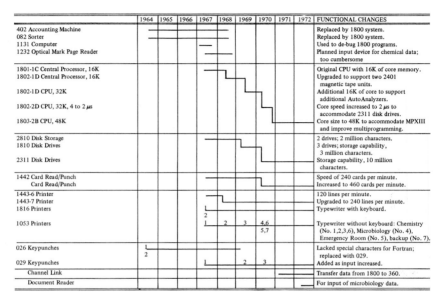

	1964	1965	1966	1967	1968	1969	1970	1971	1972	FUNCTIONAL CHANGES
402 Accounting Machine										Replaced by 1800 system.
082 Sorter										Replaced by 1800 system.
1131 Computer										Used to de-bug 1800 programs.
1232 Optical Mark Page Reader										Planned input device for chemical data; too cumbersome
1801-1C Central Processor, 16K										Original CPU with 16K of core memory.
1802-1D Central Processor, 16K										Upgraded to support two 2401 magnetic tape units.
1802-1D CPU, 32K										Additional 16K of core to support additional AutoAnalyzers.
1802-2D CPU, 32K, 4 to 2 μs										Core speed increased to 2 μs to accommodate 2311 disk drives.
1803-2B CPU, 48K										Core size to 48K to accommodate MPXIII and improve multiprogramming.
2810 Disk Storage										2 drives; 2 million characters.
1810 Disk Drives										3 drives; storage capability, 3 million characters.
2311 Disk Drives										Storage capability, 10 million characters.
1442 Card Read/Punch										Speed of 240 cards per minute.
Card Read/Punch										Increased to 460 cards per minute.
1443-6 Printer										120 lines per minute.
1443-7 Printer										Upgraded to 240 lines per minute.
1816 Printers										Typewriter with keyboard.
1053 Printers				2 / 1	2	3	4,6 / 5,7			Typewriter without keyboard: Chemistry (No. 1,2,3,6), Microbiology (No. 4), Emergency Room (No. 5), backup (No. 7).
026 Keypunches	1 / 2									Lacked special characters for Fortran; replaced with 029.
029 Keypunches				1		2	3			Added as input increased.
Channel Link										Transfer data from 1800 to 360.
Document Reader										For input of microbiology data.

date the 2311 disk drives. Finally, early in 1971, the core size was increased once again to the present configuration of 48K in order to accommodate the MPX III multiprogramming system.

CHANGES IN STORAGE CAPABILITY

Concurrent with upgrading of core size was the gradual growth of the storage capabilities of the system. In 1967, we started with two drives of the 2310 disks that had a storage capacity for two million characters. By 1969, with increased need, three 1810 disk drives were installed, capable of storing three million characters. Finally, early in 1970, the 2311 disk drives were installed, each capable of storing ten million characters. Provided that we transfer data to the files of the Medical Center computer, the present configuration will be adequate for the forseeable future.

INPUT AND OUTPUT DEVICES

Our original 1443-6 printer produced 120 lines per minute. In 1968, this was upgraded to a 1443-7 printer capable of printing

240 lines per minute. The need for typewriters and keypunches has increased steadily over the years (Table I).

LINKAGE OF THE LABORATORY COMPUTER TO THE MEDICAL CENTER COMPUTER

The channel link between the laboratory computer and the Medical Center computer (IBM 360) was installed early in 1971, for the purpose of transmiting all laboratory data from the 1800 file which is accession-number oriented to a file in the 360 which is patient-oriented.

A document reader was acquired early in 1972 for the purpose of inputting data from the Microbiology laboratory.

The capabilities of the system for input, storage, processing, and output have all been upgraded as the need arose. Each modification required some changes in the system which were unique for this laboratory and which required custom systems design and programming. In addition, it was necessary to design and build special purpose hardware, such as the process interrupt, the digital input device, and HOTC. It would have been extremely difficult for us to have accomplished this without a resident staff which was familiar with our laboratory system as well as with computer programming and engineering. It is for this reason that we do not recommend that any laboratory rely so much on the manufacturers as to purchase a *turn-key* system.

●●●●●●●●●●●●●●●●●●●●●●●●●●●

CHAPTER IX

THE RELIABILITY OF THE SYSTEM

T HE CENTRAL LABORATORY 1800 process control monitor system went on-line in October, 1968. Our objective has been to
keep the system in continuous operation twenty-four hours a day,
seven days a week. We have met this objective. The computer,
however, is an electromechanical device which does require some
preventive maintenance. In addition, from time to time there is
need to use the computer exclusively for other purposes. These
are *downtimes* which are scheduled in advance. The other cate-
gory of downtime is unscheduled and due to machine failure.

SCHEDULED DOWNTIME

Each Friday morning the system is down for two hours while
the customer engineer checks the computer hardware. During
this time the technologists perform *preventive maintenance* on
their instruments. Any emergency laboratory work during this
period is performed *off-line* and the results are calculated manually. These results are entered into the computer system as soon as
it is up again.

The computer is scheduled to be down when there is need to
test new programs or to copy information from one disk to another. Such work is usually performed between 12 midnight and
8 a.m. when there is least disruption of the laboratory routine.

UNSCHEDULED DOWNTIME

Machine failures affect our system in different ways depending
upon the unit involved and the length of time that it is down.
The on-line collection of data and the inquiry systems are seriously compromised only when the failure is in the central processing

unit or the disk drives. When this happens, data from the instruments which are on-line are lost and the technologist is forced to do some calculations by hand. When typewriter malfunction occurs, the technologist is inconvenienced but there is no loss of information, since the message is automatically switched to another typewriter. Failure of output devices, such as the line printer and the card reader, has occasionally delayed the printing of reports and other operations in the computer room but it has only rarely forced us to resort to the manual reporting of results.

NATURE OF THE FAILURES

During a period of three years, the *central processing unit* has failed on only two occasions, the longer downtime being 2.8 hours (Table II).

Table II

THE RELIABILITY OF THE LABORATORY COMPUTER SYSTEM HARDWARE

Unit	Number of Failures	Downtime (Hrs.) Average	Maximum
Central processing unit	2	1.5	2.8
Disk drives	3	6.0	8.5
Card reader	15	1.2	4.0
Line printer	31	1.5	4.0
Typewriter	109		

Observations made between January, 1970, through December, 1972.

The *disk drives* have been down longer than five minutes on three occasions. Only once have they been down long enough to force us to send out handwritten reports. To be sure, about once every two months, a transitory power failure or disk data errors have caused the disks to be inoperative for short periods. These errors have been readily correctable.

Failures in the *I/O devices*—the *card reader* and the *line printer*—have been more frequent and have delayed operations within the computer room. However, reports have been delayed longer than thirty minutes because of such failures on only five occasions and never has it been necessary to resort to manual reporting.

The six *typewriters* in the system have given us sufficient trouble that we acquired a spare one in September, 1970. Now a defective unit is replaced immediately with the spare. The customer engineer then repairs the faulty unit at his convenience.

CUSTOMER ENGINEERING SUPPORT

IBM has given us excellent service. On the average, a customer engineer has been in the laboratory within forty-five minutes after we telephoned for help.

CHAPTER X

THE COSTS

UNIT RECORD SYSTEM

T HE TOTAL COST OF RENTING the hardware for the 402 system was $16,922; the maximum annual expenditure was $4,618 (Table III). The personnel costs for development were annually in the range of $5,000 to $6,500 (Table IV). The cost of the clerical personnel for the operation of the system amounted to about $7,000 annually; that for supplies, $700. The total direct cost (hardware plus software) attributable to the 402 system was less than 4 percent of the total budget of the Central Laboratory (Table V).

1800 SYSTEM DURING THE DEVELOPMENTAL PHASE

The costs rose abruptly as soon as a decision was made to implement the 1800 system. The abortive attempt to adopt the 1232 optical mark page reader cost a total of $8,636 for rental of the hardware. The personnel costs for systems analysis, design and programming was $27,490 during fiscal year 1967-1968 and reached a maximum figure of $30,650 the following year. During 1967-1968, the cost of personnel for design and fabrication of special hardware devices was $11,650 (Table IV); it reached a maximum of $19,200 in 1970-1971; the cumulative cost to date has been $74,110. The cost of material for the special input devices has totaled to date $36,546 (Table III).

We began leasing the 1800 hardware during 1967-1968. During this year the cost was $49,320, increasing to $70,341 in 1969-1970. In October, 1969, the decision was made to purchase the system, since the IBM sales representative calculated that purchase would actually reduce the monthly payments as well as resulting in eventual discontinuation of the payments. The ex-

Table III

THE COST OF HARDWARE, MAINTENANCE, AND SUPPLIES

	FISCAL YEARS											
	1964–1965	1965–1966	1966–1967	1967–1968	1968–1969	1969–1970	1970–1971	1971–1972	1972–1973	1973–1974	1974–1975	Total
Hardware												
402 System	1,154	4,618	4,618	4,618	1,914							16,922
1131 System		3,540										3,540
1232 Optical Mark Page			1,364	5,454	1,818							8,636
Pre-1800 Subtotal	1,154	4,618	9,522	10,072	3,732							29,098
1800 System				49,320	70,395	70,341	80,135	80,994	73,215	70,263	38,294	532,957
Hardware Total	1,154	4,618	9,522	59,392	74,127	70,341	80,135	80,994	73,215	70,263	38,294	562,055
Transportation & Installation			1,139		1,155		4,752	573				7,619
Miscellaneous Equipment & Prototypes			14,277		5,000	5,000	9,769	2,500				36,546
Maintenance						3,020	11,765	13,060	13,236	(13,250)	(13,250)	67,581
Supplies (cards, forms, etc.)	200	700	700	1,000	2,000	2,000	2,794	11,222	8,265	(10,000)	(10,000)	48,881
Grand Total	1,354	5,318	25,638	60,392	82,282	80,361	109,215	108,349	94,716	93,513	61,544	722,682

( ) = Projections included in total. Purchase payments on hardware started in October, 1969, with completion in 1975.

Table IV

THE PERSONNEL COSTS FOR SYSTEMS DESIGN AND

OPERATION OF THE CENTRAL LABORATORY 1800 SYSTEM

| | | FISCAL YEARS | | | | | | | | |
		1964-1965	1965-1966	1966-1967	1967-1968	1968-1969	1969-1970	1970-1971	1971-1972	1972-1973	Total
DEVELOPMENT	Systems Analysis, Design and Programming	4,000	2,300	8,590	27,490	30,650	22,505	23,880	23,080	16,660	159,155
	Hardware Design and Fabrication				11,650	12,160	13,100	19,200	17,000	1,000	74,110
	Education	2,500	2,750								5,250
	SUBTOTAL	6,500	5,050	8,590	39,140	42,810	35,605	43,080	40,080	17,660	238,515*
OPERATIONS	Clerical Personnel	2,340	6,720	7,080	7,380	12,330	12,600	18,360	21,150	23,560	111,520
	YEARLY TOTAL	8,840	11,770	15,670	46,520	55,140	48,205	61,440	61,230	41,220	350,035

*Represents 51,000 man hours @ $4.68/hr, or approximately 25 man years.

Table V

THE RELATIONSHIP OF EXPENDITURE FOR THE

DEVELOPMENT OF THE 1800 LABORATORY SYSTEM

TO THE TOTAL ANNUAL EXPENDITURE

| | FISCAL YEARS | | | | | | | | |
	1964–1965	1965–1966	1966–1967	1967–1968	1968–1969	1969–1970	1970–1971	1971–1972	Total
Total Central Laboratory Expenditure	403,241	448,701	527,884	687,281	888,026	1,009,102	1,139,439	1,250,238	6,353,912
Cost of Hardware	1,354	5,318	25,638	60,392	82,282	80,361	109,215	108,349	472,909
Cost of Software	8,840	11,770	15,670	46,520	55,140	48,205	61,440	61,230	308,815
(% of Hardware Cost)	653	221	61	77	67	60	56	57	65
Hardware + Software Costs as % of Total Laboratory Cost	2.5	3.8	7.8	15.6	15.5	12.7	15.0	13.6	12.3

penditures of $80,135 in 1970-1971 and of $80,994 in 1971-1972 include lump sum down payments made during these periods as various components were purchased at the time that the hardware was upgraded.

When we made the decision to purchase the equipment, we innocently incurred the additional expense of about $1,000 per month for preventive maintenance. The need for supplies has risen progressively to $700 to $800 per month. As the system developed, additional clerical personnel were required to staff for additional functions and longer hours. The cost of clerical operations has risen from $7,380 in fiscal 1967-1968 to $23,560 for the present fiscal year.

TOTAL COST OF THE LABORATORY SYSTEM

The *total cost of personnel* for systems development to date is $159,155 (Table IV); for hardware design and fabrication, $74,110. Adding a sum of $5,250 for education, the total cost of personnel for systems development is $238,515. Personnel costs for clerical operation of the systems total $111,520. The total cost of personnel is $350,035.

The *hardware* for the 1800 system will have cost a total of $532,957 by the time the final payments are completed during fiscal year 1974-1975 (Table III). Transportation charges, the cost of preventive maintenance and of supplies increases the total systems hardware cost to $722,682.

The *total direct cost* of the hardware and the software for evolving and operating our 1800 clinical laboratory system is $1,072,717.

Since 1967, the *annual budget* for the hardware and the software has been between $108,000 and $170,000 (Table III, V); this represents a commitment of 12.7 to 15.6 percent of the annual budget of the Central Laboratory. The total software cost of $350,035 is 48 percent of the total hardware cost of $722,682, or 33 percent of the total cost for developing the system. This personnel cost through 1973 is equivalent to 51,000 man hours or approximately twenty-five man years of effort.

• •

CHAPTER XI

THE COST EFFECTIVENESS
OF THE SYSTEM

THE TOTAL WORKLOAD for the Central Laboratory has increased exponentially since 1964 at the rate of 18 percent per year (Table VI), more than doubling in five years.

PERSONNEL

There were 52.25 full time employees (FTE) working in the Central Laboratory during fiscal year 1964-1965, including medical technologists, laboratory technicians, clerks, and secretaries. The number of tests performed per FTE during fiscal year 1964-1965 was 6,197. If the efficiency had remained at this level during the ensuing years, the laboratory would have required 126 FTE's during fiscal year 1971-1972. A staff of this size could not have been accommodated in the available facilities. Automation and computerization have indeed reduced the need for personnel so that we had a total of 67.45 FTE's during fiscal year 1971-1972. The test/FTE ratio has increased progressively every year to the present value of 11,560, almost double the value in 1964-1965. Stated in another way, the Central Laboratory staff was almost twice as efficient during the past fiscal year as in fiscal year 1964-1965.

Although the budget for salaries more than doubled between 1964 and 1972, the personnel cost per test dropped from $0.70 during fiscal year 1964-1965 to $0.64 during fiscal year 1971-1972. When this value is adjusted with the Consumer Price Index, the personnel cost per test has actually decreased 30 percent to $0.48. Each test is requiring less personnel time.

During the eight year period between 1964 and 1972, the *total expenditure* in the Central Laboratory trebled from

Table VI

ANALYSIS OF THE WORKLOAD, PERSONNEL, AND EXPENDITURE

DURING THE PERIOD OF COMPUTERIZATION OF THE

CENTRAL LABORATORY

		FISCAL YEAR							
		1964–1965	1965–1966	1966–1967	1967–1968	1968–1969	1969–1970	1970–1971	1971–1972
CENTRAL LABORATORY	Total Workload	322,856	353,069	417,397	497,461	553,270	660,823	749,129	779,705
	Total FTE's	52.25	48.58	49.43	54.18	54.18	60.48	65.90	67.45
	Total Salaries	224,842	221,317	250,862	324,587	333,651	372,205	464,197	496,940
	Tests/FTE	6,197	7,268	8,469	9,182	10,212	10,926	11,368	11,560
	Personnel Cost/Test	0.70	0.63	0.60	0.65	0.60	0.56	0.62	0.64
	(Adjusted)	(0.70)	(0.61)	(0.56)	(0.58)	(0.51)	(0.45)	(0.48)	(0.48)
	Total Expenditure	403,241	448,701	527,884	687,281	888,026	1,009,102	1,139,439	1,250,238
	Sal/Total Exp. (%)	55.8	49.3	47.5	47.2	37.6	36.9	40.7	39.8
	Cost/Test	1.22	1.27	1.27	1.38	1.61	1.53	1.52	1.63
	Adjusted	1.22	1.22	1.19	1.24	1.37	1.23	1.18	1.22
CLINICAL CHEMISTRY	Workload	107,837	132,347	164,354	199,657	228,072	266,558	316,574	323,923
	Total Salaries	58,516	72,442	84,456	109,949	123,184	127,067	167,900	169,215
	Sal/Total Exp. (%)	53.6	51.3	50.9	48.2	41.5	37.5	40.4	38.0
	Personnel Cost/Test	0.54	0.55	0.52	0.55	0.54	0.48	0.53	0.52
	(Adjusted)	(0.54)	(0.53)	(0.49)	(0.49)	(0.46)	(0.39)	(0.41)	(0.39)
	Total Expenditure	109,181	141,345	165,780	228,348	296,554	339,274	415,315	445,334
	Cost/Test	1.01	1.07	1.01	1.14	1.30	1.27	1.31	1.49
	Adjusted	1.01	1.03	0.95	1.02	1.06	1.02	1.02	1.12
	Consumer Price Index	94.9	98.5	101.0	105.7	111.6	118.1	122.4	126.6

$403,241 to $1,250,238. During fiscal year 1964-1965, salary accounted for 55.8 percent of the total expenditure; during fiscal year 1971-1972, this item was 40 percent of the total. The salary component is a decreasing portion of the total expenditure of the Central Laboratory.

UNIT COST

The overall *average cost per test* in the Central Laboratory in 1964-1965 was $1.22. Although the actual unit cost appears to have increased incrementally to $1.63 in 1972, correction with the Consumer Price Index reveals that the unit cost in 1972 was exactly what it was in 1964, $1.22. There has been no real increase in the average cost of laboratory procedures. The personnel cost per unit has decreased; therefore, the remainder is primarily the cost of supply and of automation and computerization. The present computerized system has been developed without an increase in the real cost of each test.

COMPARISON WITH CLINICAL CHEMISTRY

During fiscal year 1964-1965, the Clinical Chemistry laboratory was already highly automated. The personnel cost per test in Clinical Chemistry was $0.54, compared with $0.70 in the Central Laboratory as a whole. The average cost per test in Clinical Chemistry was $1.01, compared with $1.22 in the Central Laboratory as a whole. Comparisons for subsequent fiscal years reveal similar results. It is evident that the total cost per test, as well as the personnel cost per test, is consistently greater for the whole laboratory than for its highly automated portion.

COMPARISON WITH OTHER HOSPITALS

The Hospital Administrative Services of the American Hospital Association compares the monthly performance of each functional unit of a hospital with comparable units in other hospitals. According to the report of October, 1971, the *total laboratory tests performed per man hour* at Colorado General Hospital was 5.33, whereas the median for the previous three months for twelve other hospitals in the district was 3.64. For ninety-three other

Table VII

COMPARATIVE COSTS OF LABORATORY TESTS

	Colorado General Hospital		Comparative Medians for Previous 3 Months			
	Current Month	Previous 3 Months	District Group 130 12 Compared	State Group 780 10 Compared	National Group 950 93 Compared	Special Group 13036 9 Compared
Total Lab Tests per Man Hour	5.33	5.38	3.64	3.64	3.21	3.05
Total Lab Direct Cost per Test	1.48	1.54	1.53	1.53	1.68	2.63

Abstracted from the Hospital Administrative Services, American Hospital Association, report of October, 1971.

teaching hospitals of comparable size in the nation, this value was 3.21. The *direct cost* at Colorado General Hospital was $1.48, compared to $1.53 in the twelve district hospitals, and $1.68 for the ninety-three other teaching institutions. This latter difference of $0.20 for a workload of 780,000 tests annually would amount to $156,000.

EXPANSION OF SERVICES

The availability of automation and the computer has enabled the Central Laboratory to expand its services and its functions. During the same interval that the unit cost has been maintained at a constant level, many *new tests* have been introduced, the average cost of which is considerably higher than $1.63. Newer tests tend to be more sophisticated and to require more costly supplies and greater technical skill. Some of these new methods which have become routine procedures in our laboratory are: *in-vitro* T_3 uptake and total thyroxine, the use of atomic absorption spectrophotometry to measure calcium, magnesium and lithium, kinetic analyses of enzymes by means of an automated discrete sample analyzer,[15] analysis of serum triglyceride and of 17-ketosteroids, determination of LDH isoenzymes, measurement of immunoglobulins, and radioimmunoassays for insulin and digoxin. In addition, quality control sera are now being prepared in the laboratory.

[15]J.R. Pearson, Pinfield, E.R., and Cooper, D.: A system for computer analysis of kinetic enzyme data from a modified Beckman DSA-560. *Clin Chem, 18:*775-777, 1972.

APPENDIX III

Table VIII

INSTITUTIONS WITH IBM 1800 CLINICAL LABORATORY SYSTEMS

MACHINE CONFIGURATION

Name & Addresses	Core Size(K)	Speed μs	Tape	Disk	Card Read/Punch	Printer	Other	1053	1816	Other	Operating System	COMMENTS
1. Geisinger Med. Ctr., Danville, Pa., 17821. T.V. Mataconis	32	4		3-1810	1442	1443	Cal-Comp Plotter	1	2		MPX V3M2	
2. J. Hopkins Univ. Hosp., Baltimore, Md., 21205. W.C. Krause	32	4		3-1810	1442	1403			2		MPX	CLDAC/CLMS* (Modified version)
3. Med. Coll. of Virg., Richmond, Va., 23219. Hosp. Data Center	32	4	2-	4-		1443			2	3-2740	MPX	CLDAC/CLMS
4. Methodist Hosp., Houston, Tex., 77025. G.D. Rountree	64	2		3-2311	1442	1443		4	2	8-2260 & PDP8L	MPX	
5. N.Y. Hosp., N.Y., 10021. R.L. Engle, Jr.	32	4		3-2311	1442	1443				2260 CRTs	MPX	
6. Phila. Gen. Hosp., Phila., Pa., 14104. R. Aidenbaum & M.A. McConnell	32	4		3-1810	1442	1443			2	22-2740	TSX V3M8	CLDAC/CLMS
7. Rochester Gen. Hosp., Rochester, N.Y., 14621. J.E. Davidson	48	2	2-2401	3-2311	1442	1443		3	3	20-357	MPX V3M2	
8. St. Joseph Hosp., Phoenix, Ariz., 85013.	24	2		1810	1442		1132	1	1		MPX	
9. St. Luke's Hosp., Milwaukee, Wis., 53215. R. Clark	24	4		3-1810	1442	1443		2	1	2-1092	MPX	
10. St. Luke's Meth. Hosp., Cedar Rapids, Iowa, 52402. L.L. Robbins	32	4		3-1810	1442	1443		3	1	16-2260	MPX V3M2	
11. St. Vincent Med. Ctr., N.Y., 10011. J.K. Moore	48	2		2-2311	1442	1443		2	1	3-Hazeltine 2000 & 2-TTY	MPX V3M2	
12. Univ. Colorado Central Lab.	48	2	2-2401	2-2311	1442	1443		1	2		MPX	
13. Univ. Mich. Hosp., Ann Arbor, Mich., 48104. T. Swanson	40	2		2-2311	1442	1443		3		3270	MPX	
14. Univ. Okla. Hlth. Sci., Okla. City, Okla., 73106. J.R. Sherburn	40	2	2-2402	3-1810	1442	1403				4-1092	MPX	
15. V.A. Hosp., Boston, Mass. E. Boling	32	2		2-2311	1442	1443	Pnch Paper Tape			8-Bunker Ramo CRTs 13 TTY	MPX	

*Clinical laboratory data acquisition system/clinical laboratory management system.

Data gathered by Dr. Garth L. Olde, Director, Division of Computer Resources and Services, University of Kentucky Medical Center, Lexington, Kentucky, 40506. Used with his permission.

In addition, we know that there is an 1800 system in the laboratory of the Little Company of Mary Hospital, 2800 West 95th Street, Evergreen Park, Illinois, 60642. Contact Mr. Richard Odwazny.

In 1964, *staff coverage* of the laboratory was from 8 a.m. to 12 midnight. Between 12 midnight and 8 a.m. only emergency services were offered on an on-call basis. The Hematology and Chemistry sections have recently been staffed twenty-four hours a day by the regular staff in rotation, thus assuring the same quality of work by the same methods around the clock.

Since 1969, the same staff has been performing venipunctures to procure specimens from hospitalized patients every morning.

OTHER BENEFITS

The availability of the 1800 system has enabled us to establish an extensive *inventory system*. A specified amount of any item which is consumed in considerable quantities is kept in stock and rotated. A code identifies each stock item. The computer periodically prints a purchase request showing stock number, description, unit price, and total price for each item, then lists this information according to vendor.

The Clinical Chemistry laboratory uses a computerized program for *scheduling of personnel* at least six months in advance.

Monthly tallies are generated automatically for both the traditional test count and the new workload recording system of the College of American Pathologists.

The Central Laboratory assists the Medical Clinic with collection of medical historical information for a *multiphasic screening program*. Cards containing questions answered *Yes* by the patient are processed with the 1800 and a summary is printed in acceptable prose according to organ systems.

The unique local financial reimbursement system for ancillary fees has enabled the Central Laboratory to contribute in excess of six million dollars to the Faculty Practice Fund since 1964.

CONCLUSIONS

Automation and computerization have reduced the need for technical personnel in the Central Laboratory. Although it has not reduced the unit cost, all of the costs for development and implementation of the computer system have been borne without research support. Accuracy and precision of the analyses have been improved and, hence, the quality of the work. The analyses are being performed with the same degree of accuracy and precision at any time of the day or night and with a more rapid turnaround time than previously. The data processing capabilities have improved legibility, storage, and retrieval of information. The availability of the computer has resulted in an improvement in the fiscal management in the laboratory. Most important of all has been the intangible benefit of the increase in the pride of the laboratory staff. The awareness of being a leader in the development of a system for the health care organization of the future has contributed immeasurably to improving morale. Our staff has gained valuable education and experience in systems analysis, programming and management, all of which will be essential for future progress in the clinical laboratory and for expansion and extension of data processing to other areas of the hospital.

●●●●●●●●●●●●●●●●●●●●●●●●●●●●

CHAPTER XII

DISCUSSION

AN EVALUATION

W E HAVE RELATED in considerable detail the planning, development, implementation, and evolution of an automated-computerized process control and data processing system in one clinical laboratory in a particular setting at a specific time. We are well aware that these sets of circumstances probably will not recur, so that whatever success that we may have enjoyed is due as much to luck as to serendipity.

The development of this system has required the unqualified support of the hospital administration and the dedicated efforts of a heterogeneous team. The ultimate test of a computer system is whether it performs the functions for which it was designed: our 1800 laboratory system works for us. It has fulfilled the objectives for which it was designed.

Technological changes can be expensive. Genuine progress has been made when such changes can be made without additional costs and result in increased productivity, improved efficiency of scarce personnel, and improved quality of care. Documenting such an accomplishment requires an honest and rigorous effort at evaluation. We have attempted to do just that and have found it to be extremely difficult. Even with the considerable effort made recently to document true expenditure, the costs, particularly for systems design and implementation, tend to be hidden in the general operating expenses. Such difficulties not withstanding, we conclude that the University of Colorado 1800 clinical laboratory system is indeed cost-effective and that the considerable time and effort which have been devoted to its development have been worthwhile.

67

INEVITABILITY OF COMPUTERIZATION

When viewed in historical perspective, the developments in the clinical laboratory were inevitable and necessary for survival. A laboratory has no alternative but to mechanize and to improve the quality of its work; the first is an economic necessity and the latter is a moral obligation. Once this decision has been made to automate, then the laboratory management has taken its initial step towards a reevaluation of the traditional functions of its personnel. Medical technologists traditionally have spent most of their time in the manual performance of tests. Since it has been demonstrated beyond a shadow of any doubt that mechanization can improve the efficiency of the analytic procedure itself at least ten-fold over the manual methods, the role of the medical technologist becomes one of a trouble-shooter and a manager of a mechanized analytic system. If this is the case, there obviously must be some changes made in the educational program to better train students for this new role.

Systems analysis as a tool in the solution of problems in the health care field is a recent innovation. As we automated extensively in the clinical chemistry laboratory, we became aware of the burden of processing the data. In adapting the 402 unit record system to our data processing requirements, we unknowingly at first, became acquainted with the elements of systems analysis. Once we had made the decision to install a dedicated laboratory computer system, we were forced to probe deeper into the subject.

We have already summarized in Chapter III the essential functions and responsibilities of the clinical laboratory. The initial step is the procurement of a specimen in the prescribed manner and with positive identification; the former is a management problem involving proper delegation of responsibility to adequately trained individuals and the latter is a problem yet to be solved by technology but in truth one which is soluble. The problem of the performance of the analytic procedure has already been partially solved by coupling automation to process control with a computer. Input, initial evaluation and comparison of data, storage, and retrieval are functions best delegated to the computer. Viewed in this perspective, the clinical chemistry laboratory is already a process-controlled data collection factory.

Some would argue that the results of this sytems analysis need not necessarily apply to hematology and to microbiology. However, our analysis indicates that already one-half of the routine workload in hematology is automated with the Coulter S counter. Before too long this instrument will be inputting data on-line into the 1800 and, hence, the process would not differ in any respect from the analytic procedure in clinical chemistry. We have not yet eliminated the trained hands and eyes of the medical technologist in the examination of the urinary sediment and the evaluation of the peripheral blood smear, but there are already in existence experimental models of instruments capable of pattern recognition and discrimination of color and size of particles. It is but a matter of time before the hematology laboratory also will become a process-controlled factory.

What then about microbiology? If the diagnostic procedures in this area are continued in the traditional manner, there is very little prospect of automation of the analytic procedure itself. However, we are already reaping the benefits of computerized data processing in this laboratory. The solution in microbiology is to adapt known automatable immunologic procedures to the technology of process control.

CLINICAL LABORATORY OF THE FUTURE

The day is rapidly approaching when technology will have advanced to the point that medical and allied health personnel will no longer be needed in the clinical laboratory, since the traditional responsibilities of these personnel will be taken over by process control computers and engineers. Specimens will be received in the engineering laboratory in containers with patient identification in machine-readable form. This identification will be read automatically and put into the computer at the instant that the chemical analysis is performed automatically in the original container. There will no longer be need to assign arbitrary accession numbers to samples or to prepare multiple aliquots.

The ideal system would provide for the continual maintenance of quality control by a feedback loop in the analytic process. The system would require microliter quantities of specimens for each analysis. Provided that the analytic system is judged by the computer to be within acceptable control limits, test information would be stored directly in a clinical data file in a computer, to which inquiry could be addressed from a remote terminal. At the present time the weakest link in the system is the lack of a fool-proof transportation and communication system to insure that the laboratory information reaches the clinician. In the ideal system there will be central storage of all clinical data with inquiry stations throughout the medical center.

With further technological advances, the laboratory will become a micro-miniaturized, feed-back, automated-process-controlled, self regulating system requiring the services of a process control engineer. With ultimate success, there will be minimal need for the present staff and their functions in the clinical chemistry laboratory. We would have reached the utopian dream of complete delegation of responsibilities to automation and the computer and almost complete elimination of the human element in the equation. Is there any doubt that there will be minimal need in this system for clinical pathologists or medical technologists in the traditional sense?

PERSONNEL REQUIREMENTS

The senior author has been interested for several years in the development of Allied Health personnel. Therefore, early in the planning for reorganization of the laboratory, one of the goals was to determine how much of the traditional responsibilities of physicians in the clinical laboratory can be delegated safely to qualified Allied Health personnel as well as to instruments and to a computer. Since there is now only one physician currently involved full-time in the Central Laboratory and since there are sixty-seven other full-time employees in this laboratory, the ratio of M.D. to allied health personnel in 1/67. We have perhaps already achieved the maximum in delegation of responsibility, since it is extremely doubtful that the laboratory could function without at least one physician in charge. The fact is that an M.D. clinical pathologist in the traditional sense is no longer required in the clinical laboratory. Lest those with vested interests react violently and emotionally, we hasten to point out that this conclusion is a result of a rational systems analysis of the functions and responsibilities of the clinical laboratory and its staff.

Our experience with our system indicates that there is very little need for a physician in the management of the day-to-day functions of a clinical laboratory. The future role of the physician in the laboratory is as a consultant to the clinician in the proper use of the laboratory, as interpreter of the results, and as an educator of students in all allied health fields as well as medical students and graduate students. Such being the case, there is need for revision of the training program for laboratory physicians; they must have a better background in clinical medicine. The laboratory physician has access to the quantitative information which is essential for clinical investigation. Moreover, with his previous experience with quality control, he has better appreciation of the accuracy and the precision of this data than most clinical investigators. The recent developments in the clinical laboratory portend better prospective design of clinical studies, provided the capabilities of the system are appreciated. The latter is a matter of education.

UNFINISHED TASKS

There is need for additional efforts in our clinical laboratory towards completion of the task of inputting *all* laboratory information into one central file. Our current file is built according to accession numbers. It would be reasonable to restructure this file by name and hospital number so that the laboratory data could serve as the beginning of a readily retrievable clinical data bank which is coupled to the demographic and financial records of the patient. We plan to accomplish this by periodically transferring data from the disk file of the laboratory computer to the disk file of the Medical Center computer by means of the channel link. Cathode ray tubes and typewriters situated throughout the Medical Center will then be used as the means for direct inquiry into

the master patient file. Our target date for establishing a prototype is July 1, 1974.

The secret of the success of our system has been total involvement of our staff and the support of a hospital administration
which allowed us considerable latitude in planning and implementation. Perusal of Figure 4 will indicate that the system grew
in a modular fashion with upgrading of the computer hardware
as the need arose. Such an approach could not have been possible
if we had contracted for a *turn-key* system and had lacked internal programming capability. Obviously we therefore cannot
agree with the recommendations of others to wait for a fully developed laboratory computer system.

REGIONAL LABORATORIES

The question is: What is the best organizational structure that
will allow a laboratory to operate continuously, give quality
service rapidly at the lowest cost, standardize laboratory procedures in the entire area, and enable it to maintain a professional
staff capable of continually upgrading the quality of the service
as well as contributing to education and applied research? With
the availability of more and more sophisticated and expensive
automated equipment and computerized laboratory systems, it
makes no sense to duplicate these facilities in each hospital. One
logical solution would be to establish *regional non-profit service
laboratories* as an integral part of the health care system. Such an
organization would maximize efficiency by the economy of scale,
reduce cost, and standardize the analytic process. It would operate
twenty-four hours a day seven days a week. It could serve as the
regional referral center for exotic and sophisticated analyses as
well as being the focus for education and applied research.

THE COMPUTER IN CLINICAL MEDICINE

There are several other areas in clinical medicine where
automation and computerization have already been applied to
the delivery of health care: electrocardiograms are being screened
by a computer; coronary care units are being increasingly mechanized and some preliminary studies have been reported on the

use of the computer to supply predictive information. Patients are being monitored with a computer during surgery and post-operatively. Computers are being used to calculate and monitor radiation dosage in the therapy of cancer and for data collection and analysis in nuclear medicine.

Clinical data collection in another guise—multiphasic screening—is becoming increasingly popular. Its acceptance implies a delegation by the physician of additional data-gathering responsibilities to allied health personnel, the automated devices and the computer, as well as a change in the traditional sequence of action in the care of acutely ill patients (Fig. 14). The traditional pattern of care of a single acute episode of illness is for the patient to voluntarily seek the assistance of the physician. The physician meets with the patient and, in the course of an hour or so, he obtains information about the past history and the present illness; he performs a physical examination, and he records all of this information manually. He then makes a presumptive diagnosis. Next he seeks the assistance of the laboratory for confirmation of this diagnosis. Depending upon the results of the initial laboratory examinations, he may request additional laboratory examinations. As a result of the synthesis of all of this information, he eventually arrives at a diagnosis and begins therapy.

With the advent of multiphasic screening, which is heavily dependent upon computer technology, data are collected before the patient even sees the physician (Fig. 15). This procedure would tend to shorten the lag between the first examination and confirmation of the diagnosis and initiation of therapy. Since these data are gathered in a definite format, the computer can be programmed to analyze and to retrieve all or any portion of the record.

The computer, when properly programmed, has an incredible capacity for gathering, storing, analyzing, and retrieving data. These data may be numerical or descriptive laboratory data, medical history, records of therapy, nurses' notes, physicians' progress reports, business administrative information, dietary orders and records, operative notes, etc. Such data are currently being collected and stored in the medical record in a haphazard manner.

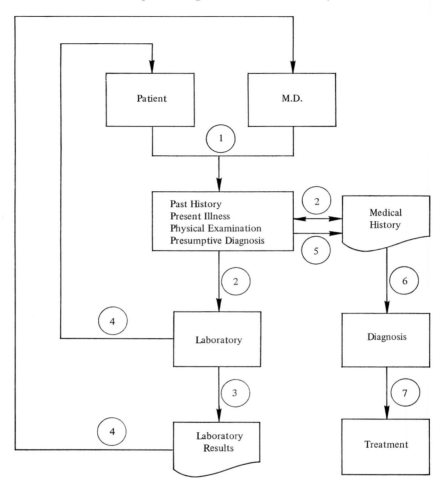

Figure 14. A schematic diagram of the traditional management of a single episode of illness.

With proper design and organization, all of this information can be gathered, stored, and retrieved as necessary with the aid of the computer. This order in the medical record can only be achieved, however, if the health team can agree upon the format and the content of the information to be stored. It should be emphasized that the computer hardware can and will store data in any form

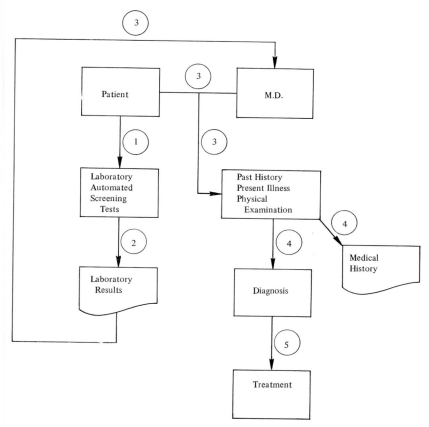

Figure 15. A schematic diagram of the proposed management of a single episode of illness.

presented to it. The dictum in computer circles states: "Garbage in, garbage out." It is the responsibility of medicine immediately and urgently to revise the data collection mechanism in order to bring order to the medical record. This effort, of necessity, must incorporate the systems analysis approach. There are some difficult decisions and compromises to be agreed upon. Since data storage can be exhorbitantly expensive, we must agree upon the minimum data content necessary to render the best affordable health care. Data collection must be made temporally more systematic and in a previously agreed-upon format. The system must be flexible enough so that modifications can be made in the future. Once begun, feed-back mechanisms could be programmed for self-improvement.

CONCERNING AMBULATORY CARE

The availability of the computer obligates the medical profession to restructure the methods for collection of data from ambulatory patients in such a way that each individual can serve as his own control. Proper design, spacing, and collection of such data, and its storage, analysis, and retrieval, will enable the health care team to practice effective preventive medicine. Much of the responsibility in such a system can be delegated to qualified Allied Health workers on the health team. The emphasis in health care will shift towards the maintenance of good health and the quality of life rather than the detection and the treatment of illness (Fig. 16).

In an ideal health care system there would be continuity of medical record throughout the life of an individual (Fig. 17). This record would commence with the fertilization of the ovum and would be uniquely identified, perhaps with a social security number. Data would be added and the record updated throughout life. The entire medical history would be stored in a retrievable form and would be transferable from one locale to another. Safeguards would be incorporated so that all of this information would remain privileged and would be released only upon consent of the patient. It is not inconceivable that within a few years each individual would carry with him, keyed to his social security number, his entire medical history coded in the space of a plastic credit card. For the first time in the history of medicine, it would be feasible and practical to store the medical information and retrieve this information so that the medical history of an individual could be collected from birth to death. That is to say, in the words of the experimentalists, each patient could now serve as his own control. With accumulation of medical information in such a form that retrieval, analysis, and correlation are possible, imagine the potential good to be derived in application of this

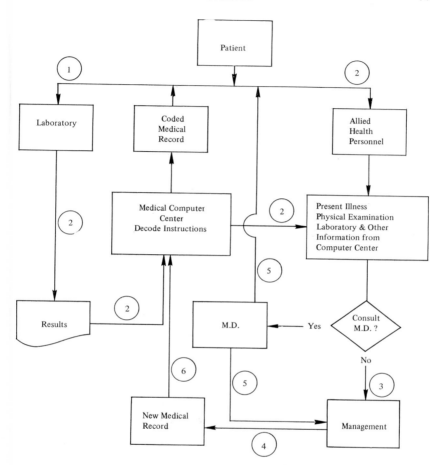

Figure 16. A schematic diagram of the preventive medical survey.

information to the preventive medical care of the individual patient.

The potential uses of such a system are limited only by one's imagination. In order that this information-retrieval system be developed to its fullest—and we have no doubt that this is a matter only of time—there exists a great need to involve clinicians in the task of standardizing the medical record. Only experienced clinicians can overcome this formidable challenge. Many of the

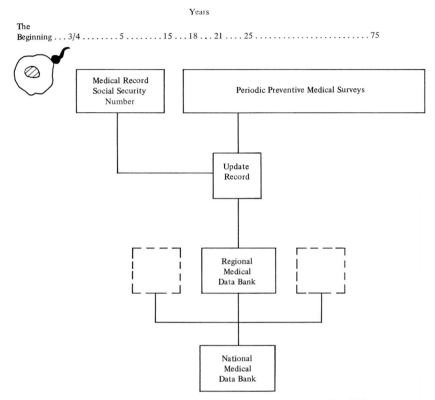

Figure 17. A schematic diagram of the future life medical history.

routine, non-medical chores of the physician will be assumed by automation and the computer. The computer hardware is already available for the establishment of regional medical centers. At least in the medical sense, it is now possible to have one world.

APPENDIX I

A GLOSSARY OF COMPUTER PIDGIN ENGLISH

Access time
: The fraction of a second required by a computer to locate and transfer a unit of data in a storage device.

Analog signal
: A continuous physical quantity or variable, such as a voltage signal from a colorimeter.

ADC
: An electronic device that converts an analog voltage signal into a digital equivalent.

Backup
: An alternate system, usually less complex or sophisticated than the main system.

Batch processing
: Accumulating and processing substantial quantities of transaction records or specimens in groups (batches).

Binary system
: A numbering system using only two symbols, which are 0 and 1.

Bit
: An abbreviation for binary digit.

Card punch
: A device that receives data in the form of electrical pulses from a computer and records them as holes in a card.

Card read/punch
: A device that both reads and punches cards.

Card reader
: A device that produces electrical pulses, corresponding to the pattern of holes in a punched card, for input to a computer.

Central processing unit (CPU)
: The controlling center of the computer which controls and supervises the entire computer system, performing the actual arithmetic and logical operations on data.

Core memory
: That component of the computer which is used for rapid random access storage and where data is stored, processed, and manipulated. Usually made of magnetic cores.

Core storage	Any storage device made up of magnetic cores.
Data processing	Manipulating data to achieve desired results.
Digital signal	Discontinuous signal, as contrasted with analog signal.
Disk storage	A form of bulk storage in which data is magnetically stored on a metal disk resembling a phonograph record. Access is rapid and storage capacity may be very great.
Downtime	Period during which a computer is not operational.
File	An organized collection of records employed in one or more data processing jobs.
Flowchart	A pictorial representation showing the sequence in which computer operations are performed.
GIGO	Garbage in, garbage out.
Hardware	The physical equipment of the computer system.
Input	The process of entering data into a computer.
Input device	A unit of a computer system which reads data into the computer.
I/O	A unit which both reads data into the computer and records processed data.
Inquiry station	A device which permits requests for specific information (stored within the computer) to be entered manually and at which the answers are printed.
Interface	The physical connection between two pieces of equipment or systems.
Interrupt	A device or program to signal the operating system to change tasks.
Line printer	An output device for high speed printing.
Machine readable	Coded to permit recognition by machine.
Magnetic disk unit	A device that can receive data from a computer and write it on magnetic disks, or read

	data from magnetic disks and transmit it to the computer.
Magnetic tape	A form of bulk storage on continuous magnetic tape.
Mark sense	An input method in which marks are machine-read directly and converted into input signals.
Multiplexer	An electronic device that allows sampling and conversion of inputs from many different devices simultaneously.
Off-line	A device or operation that is not controlled by the computer program.
On-line	Any device or operation that is directly linked to the computer and is controlled by the computer program.
On-line processing	Processing information as they occur, without accumulating batches of them.
Optical mark page reader	A device that produces electrical pulses, for input to a computer, by optically sensing penciled or printed marks on special, page-sized documents.
Output	The process of recording data that result from computer operations.
Output device	A unit that records processed data sent to it by the computer.
Pidgin	A form of expression that usually has a simplified grammar and a limited, often mixed, vocabulary; used principally for intergroup communication.
Printer	A device that receives data from a computer in the form of electrical pulses, and records them in the form of printed characters.
Program	A sequence of instructions which a computer can follow.
Programmer	A person who plans computer operations and writes computer programs.

Software   The programming instructions and commands
                            of a computer system.

Storage unit   Any device capable of retaining information.

Turn-key   The supplier assumes responsibility for fur-
                            nishing the computer, the programs, training,
                            and maintenance as a whole package. All that
                            the user theoretically does is *turn the key*.

APPENDIX II

ANNOTATED PERTINENT REFERENCES

T HE FOLLOWING are recent publications which have not been referred to in the text but which we consider to be important and relevant contributions.

COMPUTER APPLICATIONS IN THE CLINICAL LABORATORY

Anderson, N.G.: The development of automated systems for clinical and research use. *Clin Chim Acta, 25:*321-330, 1969.
> A new analytical system using centrifugal force to transfer and mix fluids in a multiple-cuvet rotor yields data signals at intervals of 3.3 milliseconds.

Ball, M.J.: An aid to diagnosis: The use of computers in automated clinical pathology laboratories. *J Med, 1:*265-298, 1970.
> A review of laboratory computer systems available in 1970 .

Brecher, G., and Loken, H.F.: The laboratory computer. Is it worth its price? *Am J Clin Path, 55:*527-540, 1971.
> Description of a PDP-8L system at the University of California Medical Center. It is recommended that any system which is found acceptable be used "as is."

Clark, F., Gross, S., and Rafferty, W.G.: Laboratory information system. *Sperry Technology, 1:*23-32, 1972.
> Description of a Sperry laboratory information system at the North Shore Hospital, Manhasset, N.Y.

Dickson, J.F., III: Automation of clinical laboratories. *Proc IEEE, 57:*1974-1987, 1969.
> An engineer discusses the social, medical, and technical considerations surrounding automation.

Gabrieli, E.R.: *Clinically Oriented Documentation of Laboratory Data.* N.Y. and London, Academic Press, 1972.
> Proceedings of a conference on subject held at Buffalo, N.Y., in May, 1971.

Grams, R.R., Johnson, E.A., and Benson, E.S.: Laboratory data analysis system: Section I—Introduction and overview. *Am J Clin Path, 58:*177-181, 1972.

The beginning of a series of articles about a system for the analysis of laboratory data.

Gray, P., and Owen, J.A.: Experience with on-line computer processing of data from an AutoAnalyzer complex. *Clin Chim Acta, 24:*389-399, 1969.
An Australian system for on-line processing using a modified sampler circuitry and a DEC PDP 8/S computer.

Johnson, J.L.: *Clinical Laboratory Systems. A Comprehensive Evaluation.* Northbrook, J. Lloyd Johnson Associates, 1971.
A survey of 97 clinical laboratory computer installations.

Levy, S.W.: The design and operation of a small computer system for the clinical laboratory. *Clin Biochem, 5:*146-158, 1972.
A Hewlett-Packard system using mark-sense cards and an optical card reader.

Linman, J.W., and Thomas, R.S.: Computerizing the blood smear report. *JAMA, 221:*1397-1401, 1972.
A light pen-video console and mark-sense cards to report blood smear interpretations.

Martin, S.P.: The clinical laboratory: Cost benefit and effectiveness. *Ann Int Med, 75:*309-310, 1971.
Have the added activity and cost generated in the clinical laboratory been associated with a commensurate benefit to the patient or with more effective care?

Melville, R.S., and Kinney, T.D.: General problems for clinical laboratory automation. *Clin Chem. 81:*26-33, 1972.
Members of the Automation in the Medical Laboratory Sciences Review Committee of the National Institute of General Medical Sciences, NIH, identify general goals for future developments.

Müllertz, S.: A system for identification and distribution of samples and for processing and storage of data in clinical chemistry. *Scand J Clin Lab Invest, 26:*407-413, 1970.
A Danish solution to the problem of sample identification, using a rubber strap.

Nelson, M.G.: Automation in the laboratory. *J Clin Path, 22:*1-10, 1969.
The Presidential address with the revised dogma given at the Annual General Meeting of the Association of Clinical Pathologists in Sept., 1968.

Payne, L.C.: *An Introduction to Medical Automation.* Phila. and Toronto, Lippincott, 1966.
A introductory text by an English pioneer at the University College Hospital in London.

Rappaport, A.E., Gemmore, W.D., and Constander, W.J.: Should the laboratory have its own computer. *Hospital Progress,* 114-124, March, 1969.
A pioneer at the Youngstown (Ohio) Hospital Association argues for a shared, off-line, batch-operated system.

Raymond, S., and Hamilton, W.F.: Clinical laboratory computers. Another point of view. *Lab Management,* 28-31, July, 1972.
> A review of the Johnson Report from the Hospital of the University of Pennsylvania.

Richterich, R., and Ehrengruber, H.: A test code for electronic data processing in the clinical chemistry laboratory. *Clin Chim Acta, 22:*417-422, 1968.
> The Swiss recommend a unidimensional, linear, six alphanumerical code.

Simpson, D., Sims, G.E., Harrison, M.I., and Whitby, L.G.: Equipment for linking the AutoAnalyzer on-line to a computer. *J Clin Path, 24:*170-176, 1971.
> Description of a British on-line system linking AutoAnalyzers to an Elliott 903 general purpose digital computer.

Straumfjord, J.V., Spraberry, M.T., Biggs, H.G., and Noto, T.A.: Electronic data processing system for clinical laboratories. *Am J Clin Path, 47:* 661-676, 1967.
> Description of an early clinical laboratory data processing system using an IBM 1401 computer.

Vermeulen, G.D., Schwab, S.V., Young, V.M., and Hsieh, R.K.C.: A computerized system for clinical microbiology. *Am J Clin Path, 57:*413-418, 1972.
> A coded, fixed data storage format for storage and retrieval of data at the USPHS Hospital, Baltimore.

Westlake, G., McKay, D.K., Surh, D., and Seligson, D.: Automatic discrete sample processing. *Clin Chem, 15:*600-610, 1969.
> Description of a clinical chemistry system using discrete sample handling and computerized data processing at the Yale-New Haven Hospital.

Westlake, G.E., and Bennington, J.L.: *Automation and Management in the Clinical Laboratory.* Baltimore, Univ. Park Press, 1972.
> Discussion of application of accounting and systems methods to the clinical laboratory, based on a conference on subject held at San Francisco, Calif., in May, 1971 .

Whitby, J.L., and Blair, J.N.: Data processing in hospital bacteriology: Experience of 18 months' trial. *J Clin Path, 25:*338-343, 1972.
> Description of a system at the Queen Elizabeth Hospital, Birmingham, England.

COMPUTER APPLICATIONS IN CLINICAL MEDICINE

Ahlvin, R.C.: Biochemical screening—a critique. *N Eng J Med, 283:*1084-1086, 1970.
> Biochemical screening is not medically justified.

Berkley, C. Editor: *Automated Multiphasic Health Testing.* New York, Engineering Foundation, 1971.

Proceedings of an international conference on engineering in medicine, automated multiphasic health testing, held in Davos, Switzerland, in Sept., 1970.

Bleich, H.L.: The computer as a consultant. *N Eng J Med, 284*:141-147, 1971.
> Description of a computer program written in MUMPS to help physicians manage patients with electrolyte and acid-base disorders.

Brunjes, S.: An anamnestic matrix toward a medical language. *Computers Biomed Res, 4*:571-584, 1971.
> A multidimensional matrix is used to record sign and symptom information.

Cochrane, A.L., and Holland, W.W.: Validation of screening procedures. *Brit Med Bull, 27:* 3-8, 1971.
> A member of the British Medical Research Council critically evaluates screening tests and their efficiency.

Collen, M.F.: Guidelines for multiphasic health checkups. *Arch Int Med, 127*:99-100, 1971.
> From the originator of the term, based on twenty years of experience.

Collen, M.F., Cutler, J.L., Siegelaub, A.B., and Cella, R.L.: Reliability of self-administered medical questionnaire. *Arch Int Med, 123*:664-681, 1969.
> A method for ranking each question according to its relative reliability.

Collen, M.F., Feldman, R., Siegelaub, A.B., and Crawford, D.: Dollar cost per positive test for automated multiphasic screening. *N Eng J Med, 283:* 459-463, 1970.
> An evaluation of the costs and the effectiveness of the Permanente automated multiphasic screening program.

Davis, L.S.: Prototype for future computer medical records. *Computers Biomed Res, 3*:539-554, 1970.
> Recommendations from a pioneer in medical methods research at the Kaiser Foundation Research Institute.

Ertel, P.Y., Pritchett, E.L.C., Chase, R.C., and Ambuel, J.P.: An outpatient data system. *JAMA, 211*:964-972, 1970.
> A computer based outpatient data system at the Children's Hospital, Columbus, Ohio.

Feinstein, A.R.: Taxonorics: I. Formulation of criteria. *Arch Int. Med, 126:* 679-693, 1970.
> Designing a format and system for coding data.

Feinstein, A.R., and Koss, N.: Computer-aided prognosis. *Arch Int Med, 127*:438-447, 1971.
> Development of procedures to use the computer to record the complete clinical course of diseases.

Feinstein, A.R., Rubinstein, J.F., and Ramshaw, W.A.: Estimating prognosis with the aid of a conversational-mode computer program. *Ann Int Med, 76*:911-921, 1972.

A stored library of coded data of the clinical course of patients with primary lung cancer can be searched for prognostic information.

Fleeson, W.P., and Wenk, R.E.: Pitfalls of mass chemical screening. *Postgrad Med, 48*:57-60, Oct. 1970.

A plea for better planning prior to widespread screening.

Fries, J.F.: Time-oriented patient records and a computer databank. *JAMA, 222*:1536-1542, 1972.

A flow-sheet format for a patient record which is computer-compatible.

Gilbert, D.B.: What possible use can computers be to medicine? *Arch Intern Med, 127*:96-98, 1971

The greatest application of the computing process to medicine and biology will be seen in the form of a stimulus to organize and define procedures and objectives rather than in the form of faster, more economical solutions.

Gordon, B.L.: Terminology and content of the medical record. *Computers Biomed Res, 3*:436-444, 1970.

A systematized medical summary using the Medical Record Form (MRF).

Gottlieb, G. L., Beers, R.F., Jr., Bernecker, C., and Samter, M.: An approach to automation of medical interviews. *Computers Biomed Res, 5*:99-107, 1972.

A standardized, common language for describing branching medical interviews.

Griner, P.F., and Liptzin, B.: Use of the laboratory in a teaching hospital. Implications for patient care, education, and hospital costs. *Ann Int Med, 75*:157-163, 1971.

Review of use of laboratory services at the University of Rochester Medical Center reveals little correlation between use of laboratory and needs of patient.

Grossman, J.H., Barnett, G.O., McGuire, M.T., and Swedlow, D.B.: Evaluation of computer-acquired patient histories. *JAMA, 215*:1286-1291, 1971.

Patients react favorably but the physicians are dubious, even though the computer performs as well as the physician.

Hershberg, P.I., Englebardt, C., Harrison, R., Rockart, J.F., and McGandy, R.B.: The medical history question as a health screening test. *Arch Int Med, 127*:266-272, 1971.

Evaluation of an automated history questionnaire used by the Lahey Clinic Foundation.

Hurst, J.W.: The problem-oriented record and the measurement of excellence. *Arch Int Med, 128*:818-819, 1971.

In support of the Weed method.

Kanner, I.F.: The programmed physical examination with or without a computer. *JAMA, 215:*1281-1285, 1971.

A pioneer describes a method using branching techniques.

Kinney, T.D., and Melville, R.S.: The clinical laboratory scientist. The use and organization of the clinical laboratory and the training of professional laboratory scientists of the future. *Lab Invest, 20:*382-397, 1969.

Proceedings of a workshop conference.

Lippmann, E.O., and Preece, J.F.: A pilot on-line data system for general practitioners. *Computers Biomed Res, 4:*390-406, 1971.

The design and implementation of an on-line medical data system for general practitioners in Exeter, Devon, England.

Lusskin, R., Korein, J., Thompson, W.A.L., and Heffernan, T.: Computer management of clinical information: Capture and retrieval of clinical orthopedic data by means of the variable-field-length format. *Bull NY Acad Med, 48:*1014-1032, 1972.

A system for capture, storage, and retrieval of orthopedic clinical information by means of keyboard devices and digital computers at the New York University Medical Center.

Mueller, W.J.: Automated system for collection and dissemination of medical information, *NY State J Med, 70:*2092-2094, 1970.

Description of a unique computer system using two satellite computers for a 300-bed hospital.

Payne, R.F.: The computer as a tool in clinical medicine. *South Med J, 64:*1216-1220, 1971.

A review of the demonstrated potential for use of computers in everyday medical practice.

Rardin, T.E.: Laboratory profile screening in family practice. A five-year study. *JAMA, 214:*1262-1268, 1970.

Analysis of 2,919 profiles secured on 1,204 patients examined in a five-year period by a family physician.

Reece, R.L., and Hobbie, R.K.: Computer evaluation of chemistry values: A reporting and diagnostic aid. *Am J Clin Path, 57:*664-675, 1972.

A computer program to display results and suggest diagnostic possibilities for 12 blood chemistry tests.

Roberts, L.B.: Partial correlation of some blood constituents. *Clin Chem, 18:*1407-1410, 1972.

Examination of correlations among some blood constituents apart from the effect of age.

Rushmer, R.F.: Accentuate the positive, A display system for clinical laboratory data. *JAMA, 206:*836-838, 1968.

A well known physiologist suggests a graphic visual display to emphasize abnormality, suppress redundancy, and reduce guesswork.

Sharp, C.L.E.H., and Keen, H.: *Presymptomatic Detection and Early Diagnosis. A Critical Appraisal.* Baltimore, Williams and Wilkins, 1968.

Numerous contributors take stock of the state of the art and discuss the value of early detection of disease.

Simborg, D.W., Macdonald, L.K., Liebman, J.S., and Musco, P.: Ward information-management system. An evaluation. *Computers Biomed Res, 5:* 484-491, 1972.

A computerized system at the Johns Hopkins Hospital increased direct patient-care activities and decreased the incidence of errors.

Swedlow, D.B., Barnett, G.O., Grossman, J.R., and Souder, D.E.: A simple programming system *(Driver)* for the creation and execution of an automated medical history. *Computer Biomed Res, 5:*90-98, 1972.

A program, which is designed for the execution of a repetitive task that is entirely data independent, directs the on-line interview and generates a narrative summary.

Thompson, H.K., Jr., and Woodbury, M.A.: Clinical data representation in multidimensional space. *Computers Biomed Res, 3:*58-73, 1970.

Use of a multidimensional spatial technique to analyze clinical data and to follow clinical course of the patient's illness.

Weed, Lawrence: *Medical Records, Medical Education, and Patient Care.* Cleveland, Western Reserve University, 1969.

The dean of the problem oriented record argues convincingly for the system.

Wilding, P., Rollason, J.G., and Robinson, D.: Patterns of change for various biochemical constituents detected in well population screening. *Clin Chim Acta, 41:*375-387, 1972.

Results from 4800 patients are analyzed.

Winkel, P., Paldam, M., Tygstrup, N. and the Copenhagen Study Group for Liver Diseases: A numerical taxonomic analysis of symptoms and signs in 400 patients with cirrhosis of the liver. *Computers Biomed Res, 3:*657-665, 1971.

A cooperative study to determine if the clinical and histologic observations in patients with biopsy-proven cirrhosis permit a meaningful classification of the patients.

COMPUTER APPLICATIONS TO MEDICAL CARE AND EDUCATION

Abrahamsson, S., Bergström, S., Larsson, K., and Tillman, S.: Danderyd Hospital computer system. II. Total regional system for medical care. *Computers Biomed Res, 3:*30-46, 1970.

Description of a real time medical information system for the total population in Stockholm.

Abrahamsson, S., and Larsson, K.: Danderyd Hospital computer system. 3. Basic software design. *Computers Biomed Res, 4:*126-140, 1971.

Details of the file structure and other components.

Atchley, D.W.: Discipline: A central issue of our times. *Arch Int Med, 124:* 761-763, 1969.
    An address concerning something essential to computerization.
Ball, M.J.: An overview of total medical information systems. *Methods Inform in Med, 10:*73-82, 1971.
    The function of a computerized medical information system as a traffic controller.
Barnett, G.O.: Computers in patient care. *N Eng J Med, 279:*1321-1327, 1968.
    Discussion of several functional areas of medical practice and the impact of computer technology upon these areas.
Caceres, C.A.: Large versus small. Single versus multiple computers. *Computers Biomed Res, 3:*445-452, 1970.
    Importance of the total medical system package.
Collen, M.F., Kidd, P.H., Feldman, R., and Cutler, J.L.: Cost analysis of a multiphasic screening program. *N Eng J Med, 280:*1043-1045, 1969.
    The Kaiser Permanente system scrutinized.
Garfield, S.R.: Multiphasic health testing and medical care as a right. *N Eng J Med, 283:*1087-1089, 1970.
    Multiphasic health testing to separate patients into the well, the asymptomatic sick, and the sick.
Laberge-Nadeau, C., Hurtubise, A., Feuvrier, M., L'Homme, P., and Soumis, F.: Projet Irodom: Informatigue et recherche opérationelle appliquées au dossier d'admission du malade. *L'Union médicale du Canada, 100:*1363-1373, 1971.
    Operations research applied to the development of a computerized hospital admission system.
Lindberg, D.A.B.: *The Computer and Medical Care.* Springfield, Thomas, 1968.
    From another pioneer.
McLachlan, G., and Shegog, R.A.: *Computers in the Service of Medicine.* London, Oxford Univ Press, 1968, Vol. I.
    The state of the art in the British Isles.
McLachlan, G., and Shegog, R.A.: *Computers in the Service of Medicine.* London, Oxford Univ Press, 1968, Vol. II.
    Systems analysis in the hospital.
Robertson, N.C., Baldwin, J.A., and Hall, D.J.: Methods of record linking. *J Chron Dis, 24:*159-169, 1971.
    Methods for matching persons and families automatically.
Schwartz, W.B.: Medicine and the computer. The promise and problems of change. *N Eng J Med, 283:*1257-1264, 1970.
    Discussion of the computer as an intellectual tool which will reshape the health care system, alter the role of the physician and allied health manpower, and change medical education.

White, K.L.: Personal health services system. Desiderata. *JAMA, 218:*1683-1689, 1971.

> A set of guidelines and a blueprint for change.

White, K.L., Murnaghan, J.H., and Gaus, C.R.: Technology and health care. *N Eng J Med, 287:*1223-1227, 1972.

> People's needs, not availability of technology, should determine policies and priorities for its application in health services.

Zammit-Tabona, V.: The WHO programme information retrieval system. *WHO Chron, 23:*295-303, 1969.

> The World Health Organization digital computer-oriented information retrieval system.

INDEX